ADVANCE PRAISE FOR

THE WELLBEING EFFECT

"Seth Serxner reminds us that wellbeing isn't a checklist—it's a living, evolving practice built on small steps, interconnected ideas, and habits that feed into one another. There's no one-size-fits-all here—Seth offers a framework that honors individuality, curiosity, and community."

— **Stephanie Szostak**, Actor and Author of *SELF!SH: Step Into a Journey of Self-Discovery to Revive Confidence, Joy, and Meaning*

"*The Wellbeing Effect* offers a powerful blueprint for anyone seeking to improve their wellbeing. With practical frameworks and evidence-based insights, it guides the reader with clarity and compassion, making the journey toward better health approachable and actionable. As someone on a 25-year wellbeing journey, I can attest to the author's discipline and authenticity. His openness in sharing the transformative impact of his personal wellbeing practices adds depth and inspiration to this timely and important book."

— **Joe Gagnon**, CEO, Ultra-Endurance Athlete and Author of *Living the High Performance Life: An Average Joe's Guide to the Extraordinary*

"This book shines a light on the robust evidence base supporting a more integrative approach to wellbeing. As someone involved the wellbeing space for many decades, I can attest to the author's discipline in walking his talk and appreciate his candor as he shares the role of wellbeing in contributing to his own health and wellbeing."

— **Kenneth R. Pelletier**, PhD, MD,
Clinical Professor of Medicine
Author of *Change Your Genes, Change Your Life:
Creating Optimal Health with the New Science of Epigenetics* and
Sound Mind, Sound Body: A New Model for Lifelong Health

"The Wellbeing Effect: Bite-Sized Practices for Busy People to Lead Healthier, Happier Lives goes well beyond the promised smorgasbord of easy-to-digest ideas on how to live our best lives. It packages a full meal of science-backed guidance into a playful tasting menu, inviting the reader to peruse a buffet of appetizing opportunities to advance wellbeing. Drawing upon his 40 years of experience as a researcher and business leader, Dr. Serxner translates heady research into clear information that is highly relatable and practical. A refreshing and engaging read for anyone interested in living life to its fullest."

— **Dr. Jessica Grossmeier**, PhD, MPH,
Author of *Reimagining Workplace Wellbeing:
Fostering a Culture of Purpose, Connection, and Transcendence*

"The Wellbeing Effect is a smart and practical approach to fit wellbeing into a busy life. This book delivers real strategies without overwhelm, and it does so with authenticity and clarity."

— **Thomas M. Chamberlain**, PharmD,
Founder & CEO, EdLogics

"What a refreshing approach to wellbeing. This book is smart, unique, and written for the busy person wanting to fit practical, health-promoting tools into their life."

— **Dexter Shurney**, MD, MBA, MPH, FACLM, DipABLM
Chief Health Officer, Blue Zones LLC
President, ACLM's Center for Lifestyle
Medicine Innovation (CLMI)

"In *The Wellbeing Effect*, author Seth Serxner writes with a curious spirit that makes personal wellbeing accessible with practical steps toward better health. A true leader in the wellbeing space, Seth not only champions these strategies—he lives them. His work has positively impacted thousands, and his book is a testament to his lifelong commitment to personal and collective wellbeing."

— **Karen Moseley**, President & CEO,
Health Enhancement Research Organization (HERO)

"*The Wellbeing Effect* offers a refreshing retake on the dime-a-dozen self-help book. In this book that is rooted in science and derived from years as an industry thought leader, Serxner serves up a substantive and meaningful guide on how to live one's best life. I highly recommend it!"

— **Laura Putnam**, Author of *Workplace Wellness that Works: 10 Steps to Infuse Well-Being and Vitality into Any Organization* and Cofounder and Chief Learning Officer of Upli

The Wellbeing Effect

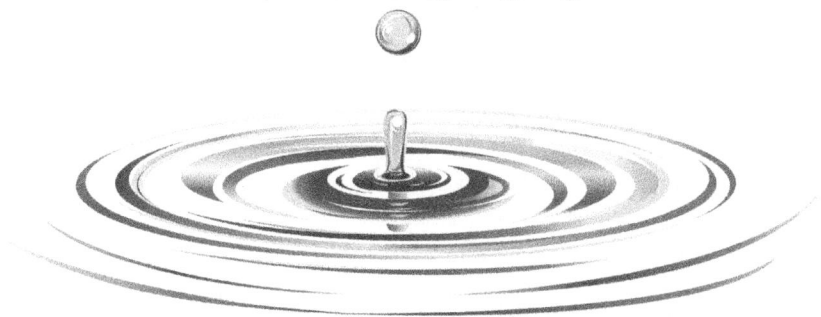

Bite-Sized Practices for Busy People to Lead Happier, Healthier Lives

DR. SETH SERXNER

modern wisdom
P R E S S

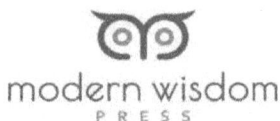

Modern Wisdom Press
Crestone, Colorado, USA
www.ModernWisdomPress.com

Published 2025

Paperback ISBN: 978-1-951692-51-3
E-book ISBN: 978-1-951692-52-0

Cover design by Toni Serofin
Back cover author photo courtesy of Siobhan Gazur
Author page photo courtesy of Michael Rosenberg

To Kari and Dayna,
the two people who are at
the core of my purpose

Contents

SECTION III
EMOTIONAL WELLBEING

Foreword

There is a tired, overused premise among many health professionals that "people already know what they're supposed to do to be healthy; they just don't do it!" It's a thinly veiled accusation that if someone suffers a health setback, they only have themselves to blame.

In *The Wellbeing Effect*, Seth Serxner explodes the myths and misunderstandings that grew out of the so-called wellness movement. But deconstructing the shortcomings of typical self-help guidelines simply serves as a launching point for this book's core purpose: serving up a rich smorgasbord of science-informed and insight-filled ideas for finding inspiration and living one's best life.

What would compel anyone to author yet another approach on what it takes to stay well, thrive, and flourish? Serxner's professional bona fides and personal stories bring us an altogether unique vantage point for helping us to appreciate that achieving wellbeing is much more accessible—and, dare I say, fun and fulfilling—than we've been led to believe.

I have worked with Seth for over 30 years, so trust me on this: You actually have three authors leading you through this journey toward self-awareness and full potential. There's Seth the Science Guy, Seth the Business Guy, and Seth the Regular Guy. In this book, Serxner shows us how what we know can shape what we do and how our goals in our work and personal lives all provide the fodder we need to fuel a fulsome existence.

As someone who has organized dozens of national health promotion conferences and think tanks, I don't use the term *thought leader* lightly. Serxner the Science Guy is one of those rare subject experts who I recruited to return often as both a main stage presenter and a panel facilitator for plenary sessions. As you will find in this book, Seth has a knack for asking the pithy questions, delving fluidly into explaining complex concepts, and astonishingly, keeping it light and laughter-filled at the same time.

I have also often sat across from Seth the Business Guy. When I was the CEO of a nationally renowned worksite wellness company, Seth was with a major consulting firm advising multinational corporations about how to best execute the employee health and wellbeing strategies he had helped them develop. His interrogations about our company's ability to deliver on health and wellbeing initiatives were always deeply informed, respectful, and refreshingly kind-spirited and light-hearted. We were all buttoned up in suits and ties, but Serxner always managed to show us how not to take ourselves too seriously.

As much as I became an admirer of Serxner's smarts and leadership in boardrooms and research roundtables, it is Seth the Regular Guy who makes this book and the guidance herein most captivating and enlightening. He relates a story about why a prestigious researcher recruited him as a research assistant. Said the professor about why he wanted Seth: "I need someone to keep me learning in a curious place, not a knowing place." It's an attitude and approach that has served Seth well as an esteemed forerunner in the field of health promotion. As a facilitator of conference panels with other business leaders and scientists, he often admonished them to "stay curious." It is his way of tempering our tendencies to proffer advice or pontificate. And it's what I enjoyed most in reading *The Wellbeing Effect*. While there are plentiful self-care tips and easy-to-try lists for making more of our moments count, this book primarily shifts our mindset to embrace what makes life most bountiful. Joy and awe come from finding and releasing our assets, says Serxner, not from reducing our risks.

Instead of nudging you toward making more goals, as if New Year's resolutions aren't burdensome enough, here is a book that has us pause to consider what matters. Serxner points out that "Wellbeing isn't a program or a product. It's just what we do and who we are." His invitation into this kind of self-reflection gives us the space to consider what it is we're hoping for in this life.

There is an old bromide that asks: "How do you eat an elephant?" The answer, of course, is "one bite at a time." And so it is with the *The Wellbeing Effect*, because it is Serxner the Regular Guy who shares his personal vulnerabilities to remind us that this book is far from a sermon on the mount. Instead, he offers up health hacks that have worked for him and others right alongside personal setbacks that have kept him humble.

The Wellbeing Effect draws as much of its authority from Seth's personal stories as from his leadership in business and academia. He reaches back to learnings from his college days to explain how "my vegetarianism is more about environmental impact than health." Decades later, the rest of the world is finally coming to just such a realization.

Perhaps it was unconscious, but Seth's choice of *The Wellbeing Effect* as a title comes remarkably close to how I and so many others in the health profession experience Seth as a person. That is, he exudes happiness, kindness, and caring, and his personal approach to wellbeing does, indeed, have an effect on others. At one point in the book, Serxner describes an informal business dinner where someone asked the group: "How do you pay it forward?" I happened to be at that dinner and remember it well. Seth, with his usual self-deprecating style, credited everyone else in the group as having save-the-world-level aspirations. But he made no mention of his seminal impact on our field.

What I love most about this book is the way it so methodically captures the many ways that Serxner has helped advance the science behind wellbeing, and how workplaces have benefitted from his wisdom and counsel. What's more, readers should know that behind the stories of those who have improved their lives are unspoken episodes where Seth has personally lifted up many others with his encouragement, wit, and good humor. He writes: "Ultimately, generosity is a way of life that includes sharing and support of others." Serxner has long been a wellbeing influencer, and his impact is far from over, but I anticipate I will often cite this book in the years ahead as a gift from Seth. Book writing is hard work, and this book is a wonderful, generous act. My thanks go out to Seth for paying it forward.

— **Dr. Paul E. Terry**

Editor-in-Chief of the *American Journal of Health Promotion*, Senior Fellow at the Health Enhancement Research Organization (HERO), Author of *Well Advised: Your Guide for Making Smart Health Decisions* and *Breaking Stone Silence: Giving Voice to AIDS Prevention in Africa*

Introduction

We plan some life-changing moments: a graduation, a wedding, a milestone birthday celebration. But most happen out of the blue, turning your world upside down in seconds.

That's how it was for me on a ski trip in Lake Tahoe with my daughter a week before Christmas 2024. Beautiful blue skies turned into a Code Blue medical emergency after a freak accident on a favorite mountain run that we'd been skiing together for over 25 years.

It all started innocently enough: I caught the inside edge of my ski, and the skis didn't release. I went down, bouncing hard on my front side, landing face-first and spread-eagle. The force of the forward impact flipped me midair onto my back, causing me to whiplash my head and crack my helmet. Lying on the ground, half-stunned and half-embarrassed, I waved off a couple of good Samaritan skiers who offered to help me get medical attention. You'd think that as a health and wellness expert, I'd know better, but shock is a powerful thing.

I continued skiing the rest of the run to the ski patrol first aid hut. After checking for a concussion or any obvious injuries, they helped me to my car, and my daughter drove me to a nearby urgent care for a CAT scan.

This is where things took a dramatic turn. Before they could hook me up, I passed out. From the waiting room, my panicked daughter heard the team announce my Code Blue status, thanks to low blood pressure, significant fractures to my pelvis, and life-threatening internal bleeding. Within minutes, we were in an ambulance, flying down the mountain highway to the nearest hospital—the longest 45 minutes of our lives.

While they took me into emergency trauma surgery to stop the bleeding, my daughter was asked to approve extreme measures should something happen during the surgery, adding to her panic and overwhelm. Thankfully, we both got lucky: The advanced directive was unnecessary, as that first surgery went well. After a brutal night in the intensive care unit (ICU), a second surgery was conducted the following day to put Humpty Dumpty's pelvis back together again in a nearly five-hour surgery—nine screws, plates, and who knows what else they put in there. I returned to the ICU for another couple of nights and spent the rest of the time on the orthopedic floor.

Finally, a week later, on Christmas Day, I was discharged. During the four-hour ride home, I realized that although everything looked familiar, nothing felt the same. And that wasn't necessarily a bad thing. This terrible accident reaffirmed for me the effect of embracing our wellbeing. If you maintain a wellbeing mindset, not only can you survive life-altering experiences, you can truly thrive.

Here's what I mean by that: As I lay in my hospital bed, I was incredibly emotional and profoundly thankful. Grateful my injuries weren't worse. Full of appreciation for the amazing doctors, nurses, and medical team caring for me. And so grateful and overwhelmed by the love and support of family, friends, and community. I cried every day, several times a day, at the kindness coming my way by text, calls, and flowers. It was like hearing my eulogy without actually dying.

As I was doted on by the nurses (who are angels in human form!), I tapped into a deep sense of human connection and marveled at our interdependence. I realized that my risk-taking actions impacted others around me in ways I could not have imagined. I saw my wife and daughter scrambling to ensure I had the care I needed, both immediately and long-term, as it would take weeks to resume the activities of daily living. My best friends, also avid skiers, were rattled, reportedly saying to each other, "If Seth could crash, then what about us?" I realized that the ripple effect of our actions is profound, and it made me rethink my behavior going forward.

As down and broken as I was, I leaned into the experience as a great lesson in being present. There is nothing like pain to put you in the moment! But really, it was an opportunity—a requirement—to slow down and be here now. A growth moment. Mindfulness became a way of life, as I had to eat slowly and taste each bite. A simple conversation with someone meant being intentional about focusing. I had to stop multitasking because I could barely do the task before me, let alone multiple things at once. Moving at all required intense concentration. Breathing was measured by a monitor that beeped if I wasn't doing it correctly.

Without being able to rely on how I always did things, I had to take on a "beginner's mind," where I saw everything as a new experience.

All told, responding to my trauma involved everything I knew about a wellbeing mindset. Being grateful, having a positive attitude, staying connected, being present and paying attention, and even keeping a sense of humor (my daughter told me that I was telling jokes on the way in and out of surgery!) were all in play. And not just those aspects of wellbeing but everything I wrote about in this book, which you're about to explore.

While I'd never wish a traumatic event on anyone, it's been my experience over the past four decades that it often takes a life-changing situation for people to focus on their health and wellbeing. At that point, it's often too late—and now that I've had my own brush with mortality, I can say from firsthand experience that having a wellbeing mindset is critical.

The good news is that the book you're holding has a mountain of information about how to lead a happier, healthier, more abundant life, all broken down into digestible, easy-to-read chapters. So no more excuses! It's time to embrace your new wellbeing mindset.

Let's dive in.

CHAPTER 1

The Evolution from Wellness to Wellbeing

By now, you know that skiing is an important part of my life. While the exercise is great, it's also become a great reason to reconnect with some of my closest friends. Every year, I go on a ski trip with friends I've known for decades. Last year, 22 of us attended our thirty-fifth trip. Originally brought together by our mutual love of skiing and the outdoors, our motley group has built unexpectedly deep bonds. Over 30-some years of hearty skiing and festivities, our conversations have shifted. In our 20s, we talked more about skiing and shared history. Now, we talk about our purpose, the importance of our social connections, our focus on staying healthy and fit, our gratitude for the life we are living, and the significance of connecting to the natural world.

I bring this up because these are some of the themes I explore in this book. My goal is to provide you with a different point of view on health and wellbeing—one that doesn't feel like it's one more thing to do on top of your already busy life. You will come to see that wellbeing is a mindset and an approach to life that is not separate from your daily living but it's at the core of how you live.

Throughout my education and career of more than 40 years, I have accumulated a perspective on health and wellbeing that I've always wanted to share. This book offers you a buffet of wellbeing concepts and ideas—some that may be familiar to you, some that are new—from which you can choose what "tastes" best to you, where you want to start, what goes best together, and how much you want to do at one time. It's designed to take off some of the pressure we all feel about the need to get healthier, lose weight, be fit, meditate, and eat better.

I also hope you take away practical tips you can apply in your life. We will address the big questions, such as these: Why bother being healthy? Is it really worth the effort? Maybe those seem basic, but the very personal answers are foundational to your unique wellbeing journey.

Let's begin by defining a few key terms. Initially, wellness and wellbeing meant the same thing, but over time and with practice, one could understand them as two different concepts. One view is that the practice of *wellness* means minimizing behaviors and lifestyles that put someone at premature risk of illness and death from conditions such as heart disease, cancer, and diabetes. Wellness research is about lowering risk. In comparison, *wellbeing* means enjoying a long, healthy, and fulfilling life. Wellbeing research identifies ideas and practices that support such a good experience. In other words, wellness is about those behaviors that can make you sick and kill you, but wellbeing is about those behaviors that help you live a high-quality life.

Another way to think about it is that wellness pursues the *quantity* of life (that is, years to live), and wellbeing pursues the *quality* of life, going beyond the physical arena to consider mental, emotional, and spiritual realms as well. Both are important and build on each other.

This book translates the science of wellbeing and brings it into the practice of everyday living. We'll focus on wellbeing rather than wellness. In the following chapters, I'll cover different scopes of wellbeing that range from *foundational* to *holistic* to *emotional.*

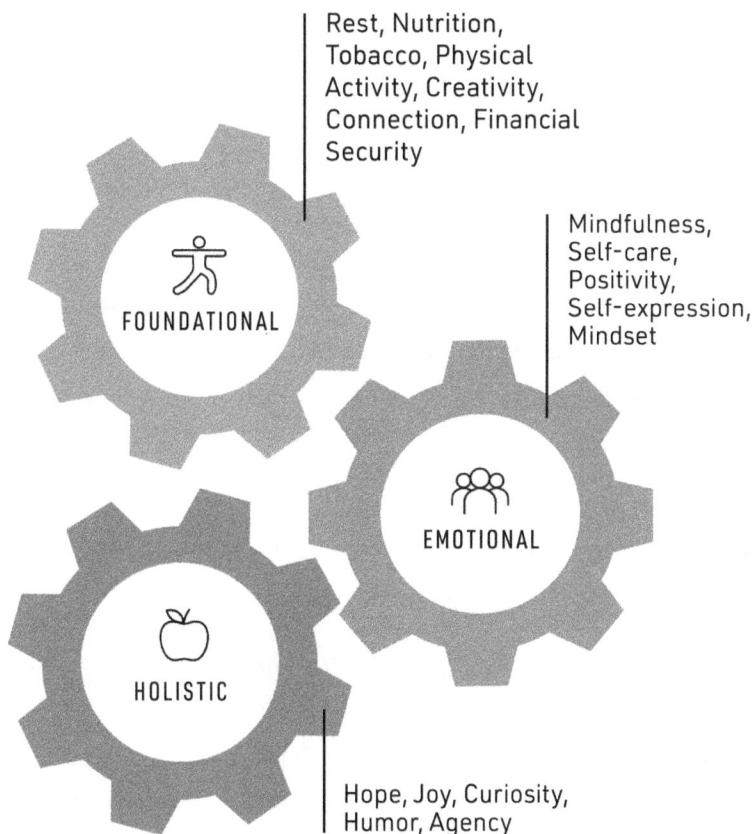

Rest, Nutrition, Tobacco, Physical Activity, Creativity, Connection, Financial Security

Mindfulness, Self-care, Positivity, Self-expression, Mindset

FOUNDATIONAL

EMOTIONAL

HOLISTIC

Hope, Joy, Curiosity, Humor, Agency

Domains of Wellbeing

Foundational wellbeing involves familiar health practices, but in this book, the focus is on your unique situation, motivation, and goals rather than one-size-fits-all advice. For example, in a wellness context, quitting smoking would be a priority lifestyle change regardless of circumstances. From a wellbeing perspective, we give more consideration to why someone smokes in the first place—is it to lose weight, relax, or even just take a break? Once we identify important personal priorities, the wellbeing mindset may lead the person who wants to quit smoking on a different path. Perhaps figuring out an approach to healthy eating, stress management, and relaxation is the first step, and then quitting smoking becomes part of the plan.

Holistic wellbeing encompasses a range of next-level ideas—including hope, humor, forgiveness, and generosity—that you can explore to enrich your life.

Finally, **emotional wellbeing** builds on that foundation by recognizing that your mental health matters, and you can cultivate it with self-care, mindfulness, mood-shifting practices, positivity, and self-expression.

Before we jump into the content of this book, here's a little personal background about how I came to be a wellbeing expert that might help you relate to the approach I'll be sharing with you.

I grew up in Southern California in the 1960s and 1970s, went to the University of California at Santa Cruz (go Banana Slugs!), and studied psychology and biology. I then got my master's degree in public health at the University of California at Los Angeles and my PhD in social ecology at the University of California at Irvine, where my research focused on health promotion and disease prevention.

When I was in graduate school, corporate wellness was just emerging as a field of study. The corporate wellness programs at the time were focused on questionnaires called Health Risk Appraisals. They asked about your weight, exercise habits, stress management, smoking, drinking, and other lifestyle topics. Then they gave you feedback about your highest-risk behaviors. All that information was intended to motivate you to make changes in your lifestyle so that 30 or 40 years in the future, you might live another year or two longer.

Let's think about that for a second. The advice at the time was to forgo the pleasure today and receive the distant, delayed gratification that you might live longer.

Is it any wonder that perspective didn't work so well? While well-intended and evidence-based in the approach, the questionnaires didn't really tell the participants anything they didn't already know. People would say, "I know I'm overweight, don't eat well, and should exercise more. Tell me something I don't know."

Since then, the wellness industry has evolved, as has the science. I've paid close attention to this evolution, and these days, I support the modern notion that *wellbeing* is the best goal for most of us to focus on. I built a 30-year career in corporate health and wellbeing, helping companies keep their employees and families healthy so they could be productive, happy, and well. Thanks to that focus, I've gotten good at translating health and wellbeing research from expert studies into clear information that regular people can use right away to enjoy their life today…not decades from now.

In the chapters ahead, I will share the lessons, themes, and insights that I acquired from my academic, corporate, and personal experiences. As I've mentioned, I think of this as a wellbeing buffet you can peruse before you make choices about what "tastes" right to you. However, there is a certain logic to the way the chapters are organized. You'll discover three main sections and themes of wellbeing in the chapters ahead: foundational, holistic, and emotional. All of these bite-sized chapters are valuable aspects to living a healthy life—in body, mind, and spirit.

However, before you start sampling the wellbeing buffet, I want to be sure you're set up to successfully make positive changes to support a healthier lifestyle and wellbeing mindset. Chapter 2 provides insight into behavior change, so you'll have the tools and confidence necessary to digest the wellbeing practices in the book and make them a part of your daily "diet."

Finally, I encourage you to use the book as a handy reference throughout your personal wellbeing journey. Enjoy yourself as you "taste test" all the concepts! As one CEO who was in favor of everything I was teaching his employees noted, "If it's not fun, they won't do it." So let's have some fun with these easy-to-implement health hacks. You deserve a life full of the positive effects of wellbeing!

CHAPTER 2

The #1 Idea to Chew On: You Can Change

I thought about putting this chapter at the end of the book because, for many, behavior change seems impossible, and that might sabotage your wellbeing journey before it even starts. So, feel free to skip ahead and come back later after you've explored the other chapters. However, whenever you choose to read this chapter on behavior change, rest assured that I'll keep things simple and relatable—starting with a few examples from back when I was growing up (about 55 years ago) that prove profound behavior change is indeed possible.

Do any of these sound familiar?

- Back when fast food was a new concept, McDonald's was all the rage. As the number of franchises grew, so did the litter. People had no place to throw away their food wrappers and drink cups, so they just tossed them out of their car windows.

- In 1965, 45% of adult Americans smoked, with even higher rates in some age groups.[1] And by the way, both my parents smoked. My mother stopped during her third pregnancy (with me) due to a horrible coughing fit, but my dad had a really hard time quitting and only stopped in his 70s.

- My favorite place in a car was the back window deck—so warm and cozy. At that time, there were no seat belts, let alone child car seats, so my friends and I just bounced around in the back of the vehicle, and the parents didn't say anything.

What do these examples have in common? All of these behaviors have significantly declined in recent decades (for example, littering has decreased by 61%,[2] only 16% of American adults smoke,[3] and in most states, at least 90% of people wear seat belts[4]). How did this happen? Here are some lessons researchers have learned from these and other changes in societal behavior.

- When used properly, mass media can educate people and encourage new behaviors. Programming that connects to personal emotions is very powerful.

- Policies and regulations—such as increased taxes, restricted access for minors, and limited advertisements—played a significant role in reducing smoking rates.[5]

- Financial incentives and fines have also contributed significantly to changing littering and seat belt habits in this country.[6]

- Surprisingly, product design influences change as well. For example, having different-colored trash and recycling bins widely available helps discourage littering and support recycling.[7]

- Peer pressure can promote both positive and negative behaviors. As the behaviors of peer groups change, individuals often tend to follow suit. In other words, if everyone is wearing a seat belt, I am more likely to wear one.

The Pyramid of Habit Change

Now, let's translate those lessons into principles you can apply to your wellbeing journey. What forces inspire a person to change? From the examples above, we can highlight pain-avoidance (such as avoiding a fine), pleasure-seeking (such as gaining a reward), awareness (that is, knowing about the need to change and why it matters), emotion, community support, convenience, and habit (for example, an easier seat belt is one that will get used).

We can then organize these motivating factors into a pyramid.

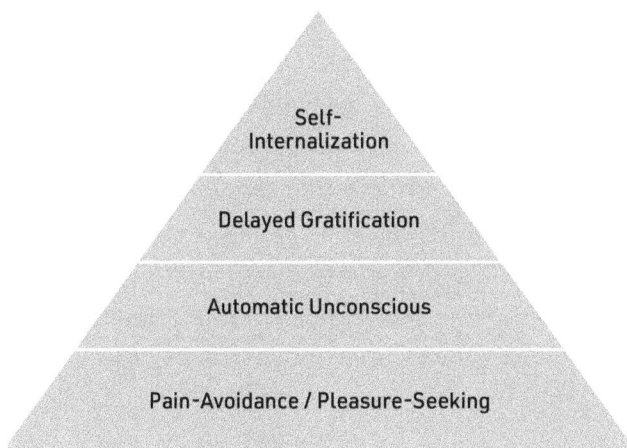

Health Behavior Models: Human Motivation

- The big foundational base consists of **pain-avoidance and pleasure-seeking**. Of course, both pleasure and pain are subjective and may vary by individual or change over time, but essentially, they are major, primal drivers of behavior. For example, peer groups provide pleasure when they offer acceptance or pain when they are exclusive.

- The next level in the pyramid focuses on **habits**. This is where behaviors become automatic. Brushing your teeth is a great example of a healthy behavior that may have started as something that feels good and is beneficial for you but eventually became a routine behavior.

- The third level is **delayed gratification**. It's the understanding that what I do today will affect the future, so if I want to avoid *future* pain or experience *future* pleasure, I may need to experience some level of pain or lack of pleasure *now*. With seat belts, for example, educational and emotional mass media helped instruct and inspire us to weigh the future benefits of safety for ourselves and our loved ones against the relatively minimal hassle of buckling up.

- The top layer of the pyramid is where behavior becomes **internalized**. An internalized behavior isn't just a routine for you—it truly feels like part of your identity. In the context of wellbeing, at this level of the pyramid, you adopt a healthy lifestyle not because you make a daily choice to do so, but because you see yourself as a healthy person. Being physically active, eating well, and getting adequate sleep are not about pain or pleasure but about who you are.

Three Steps to Achieve Lasting Personal Behavior Change

My three-step process for accomplishing individual behavior change builds on this background. Most likely, no one has ever really taught you how to systematically change your behavior. As a child, you may have been told to clean up your room, and you did it because you'd get in trouble if you didn't. Maybe you grew to like a clean room, so you internalized the benefits, but maybe not. It was all trial and error, unconscious behavior-shaping by parents, authority figures, peer groups, and the culture.

Now when you want to change a behavior (such as saving more money, eating healthier, or being more active), you end up winging it. But you don't have to. Behavior change is a process you can learn. That process has three stages: awareness, skill building, and maintenance.

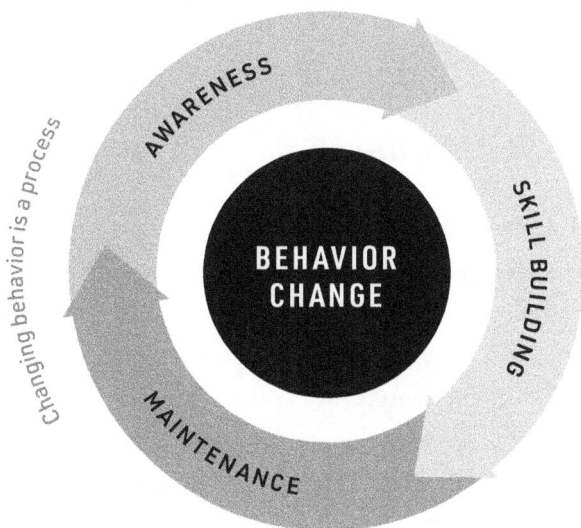

Behavior Change Framework: ASM Model - Science to Practice

Stage #1: Awareness

People often skip this stage—mainly because no one tells us we need to do it. However, it's an essential part of creating change. This is the step where you ask yourself "Why bother?" or "What's in it for me?" Behavior change can be uncomfortable and challenging, so being crystal clear about *why* you are making the change is critical to your success. As you move deeper into the process, your awareness of your motivation will support aspects of behavior change such as delayed gratification and internalization.

This phase truly revolves around *self-awareness*, which is connected to your personal sense of *purpose*. Take some time to reflect on your purpose and use it to ground yourself in the behavior-change process. Write down your findings. Remember, this process is not only a crucial step in creating behavior change; simply *having* a sense of purpose enhances wellbeing! Self-awareness is a much more powerful engine for change than "because you should" or "because your dentist told you to"!

Stage #2: Skill Building

Recently, I began playing pickleball (along with everyone else, apparently). One reason the sport has gained popularity so quickly is that it's relatively easy for most people to play. Although there is a learning curve, most players experience some success and have fun during their first attempts. Moreover, fellow players often share tips and enjoy a good laugh together; everyone makes mistakes and learns collectively. There is a satisfying sense of accomplishment. The effort is challenging, but not so difficult that success is out of reach.

The pickleball trend reflects research about how adults successfully build new skills. One of the strongest predictors of whether someone will try a new behavior is their level of confidence that they can do it successfully. If you ask someone "How confident are you in your ability to cook a delicious low-fat meal?" and their answer is "Not very," then the chances of them even trying to cook that meal are very low. Adults don't like to fail. And definitely not in public.

As an adult working to implement a new behavior, you'll need to be prepared for the rewards and setbacks that come with building a new skill. You'll want to think about ways to maximize your sense of success and remain resilient when things—inevitably—don't always go your way. Here are some ways to do this.

- **Break the new skill or behavior down into small, achievable steps.** For example, don't just tell yourself that you need to cook a healthy meal. Instead, think about the steps you can take as you have the time and energy, such as finding a recipe, making a grocery list, buying ingredients, setting out what you need... and finally, cooking! Accomplishing each of these steps is a *win*—the key to sustained learning.

- **Look for ways to make new behaviors easier.** For example, if you are trying to exercise first thing in the morning, make it easy to get dressed: sleep in some or all of your workout clothes and put your shoes and socks by the bed. These actions remove obstacles that slow you down in the morning.

- **Try different ways to learn.** People learn in various ways and at varying paces—it depends on the task at hand. Do you prefer to read directions, watch a video, or see a live demo? If one style or method of skill building isn't working for you, try another. Keep iterating, revising, and adapting your approach.

- **Make learning the new skill fun.** For example, if you want to make running a habit, you might find that jamming out to some great music helps. Look for ways to inject pleasure into the behavior change that you desire, and you will likely be successful.

Failing Upwards

Breaking the new skill into simple, achievable steps and identifying ways to make those steps easier and more fun helps satisfy our need to feel good about making progress. But what about our desire to avoid failure? In fact, failure is not a serious barrier—it's just new information that we can use on our journey.

This kind of resilient thinking is called having an "iterative mindset."[8] When you have this, it means you are in a constant mode of experimentation and discovery as you explore what works for you. If you want to start exercising regularly, you might set an initial goal to walk for 15 minutes every morning. You set the alarm, lay out your clothes, and clear your schedule—but end up sleeping in rather than facing a cold morning walk. One story you could tell yourself is "I failed—guess I'm not cut out for exercise."

However, an iterative mindset suggests a different narrative: "I think I need to redesign my approach. Maybe I'll try exercising in the afternoon. Perhaps I'll invite a friend to join me, which could make it more enjoyable and keep me accountable." You haven't failed.

Instead, you're engaged in a continuous design process to discover what works for you.

A final way to approach your skill-building process is to remember what worked for you as a kid. Adult Learning Theory recognizes that adults learn differently than children. Kids try many new things, and they fail all the time. This is expected and planned for, not treated like it's a disaster. However, adults tend to try limited things, and when they fail, they often panic and retreat.[9]

When working on your new skills, you can recognize that the way you learn as an adult is different from when you were a child. Give yourself support for that, and try to get back to the nonjudgmental, experimental mindset you likely enjoyed when you were young.

Stage #3: Maintenance

People often tell me that maintenance—transforming a new behavior into a habit, a regular aspect of your life—is the most challenging part of behavior change. I don't believe it has to be that way. The issue is that no one focuses sufficiently on maintenance! In some cases, it's because capitalist business models lack the incentive to assist you in maintaining behaviors. Instead, many of these models profit from your *failure* to maintain them.

Consider fitness gyms and nutrition supplements, which require up-front payments yet show little concern if you don't attend the gym or finish all your protein powder. Interestingly, researchers possess substantial knowledge about maintenance—we simply don't design for it. The insights gained from treating substance-use disorders and addictive behaviors can, in fact, also aid us in adopting and sustaining healthy behaviors. We understand how to help individuals quit smoking—for good—which indicates our knowledge about maintenance.

Based on all this research, I recommend the following key strategies to help you maintain your new behavior.

- **Use incentives.** As you learned in the skill-building section, it's important to experience the feeling of each small success. Incentives help you do that. These rewards don't supplant or override the underlying intrinsic motivation for the behavior (which is driven by your purpose) but are more of a bonus or a gift to yourself. For example, I'm a runner, and while I'm personally motivated to run so I can be outside in nature alone with my thoughts and do something good for my health, I also enjoy a new pair of running shoes! Every time I hit the 500-mile mark, I buy new sneakers. Consider rewards that bring you joy and will inspire you to keep going—things like exercise clothes, cookware, music, or books.

- **Anticipate and plan for failure.** As I mentioned in the skill-building section, failure is common, if not inevitable, and it offers a chance for you to fine-tune your plan. The iterative mindset remains crucial during this maintenance stage, just as it was when you began. If you miss a day of exercise or eat something you're trying to avoid, learn from the experience and consider how to adjust moving forward. Don't judge yourself; this is a long-term commitment. Stay open and curious about the process and consider how you might modify your approach in the future.

- **Create a supportive environment, both socially and physically.** Start by identifying people around you who support your goal. For example, I'm an avid cyclist who doesn't mind riding alone, but some days, in the foggy, cool, windy coast where I live, it can be a bit challenging to get out and ride. Knowing I have a crew of friends who are expecting me and will "suffer" with me is the extra motivation on those days when it can be tough to get started. Likewise, creating a physical environment to support your maintenance is also key to the process. For example, if you'd rather watch TV than exercise, add a television to your exercise space so you can stream shows while working out.

And one more important thing to consider when changing your habits: Stay hopeful. New behaviors can be challenging at first, but they get easier with repetition and practice. Over time, you'll experience a significant boost in maintenance as you start to see these behaviors as part of your identity. This happens when your perception shifts from "I run" to "I am a runner" or from "I eat healthy foods" to "I am a healthy eater." The behavior becomes internalized and ingrained in your self-image. There is no set timeframe for this change in self-identity, but it's worth striving for, even if it means practicing consciously. Once the behavior feels like an integral part of who you are, maintaining it will come naturally.

Now that you have tools for successfully changing your behavior, it's time to dig into the wellbeing buffet!

FOUNDATIONAL WELLBEING

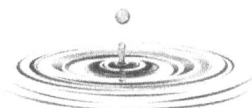

Foundational wellbeing involves providing yourself with a healthier, better-rested, more energetic body and a more stable, supportive environment. You've no doubt encountered many of the topics you'll read about in this section before, but probably in a wellness context. You'll see them in a new light when we approach them from a wellbeing perspective.

CHAPTER 3

The Art of Sleeping Well

When I first brought up the importance of sleep to corporate wellness professionals, in the early 1990s, I was literally laughed out of the room. The idea of creating "quiet rooms," not to mention "nap rooms," was out of the question. "What, you want me to pay people to sleep on the job?" one executive exclaimed.

These days, when I talk with people about health and wellbeing, getting quality sleep and feeling energized rank among their top priorities. The research is clear that adequate sleep leads to stronger decision-making, less risk-taking behaviors, better cognitive capability, improved physical health, increased attractiveness, and more energy.[1] Sleep provides an essential opportunity for the body and brain to recover, regenerate, and regroup.

During the COVID pandemic, I caught up on my sleep, and the benefits astonished me—even as a wellbeing expert! I had not realized that more than 20 years of weekly cross-country flights had thrown my body into a sleep deficit. Being in different time zones, staying up for business dinners, getting up early to try to maintain some sort of exercise routine, getting home late, and trying to catch up on the weekends had taken its toll. It took me about six months of non-travel to recover.

Wow, what a difference it made to get eight hours of sleep every night! I was more alert in meetings and had more energy. People told me that I looked well rested. Even since the pandemic, I have worked to maintain a good sleep schedule, and when I do travel, I prioritize sleep over early-morning meetings.

Prioritizing rest and relaxation can be hard for some personality types—clearly, I'm one of them. My college roommates would make fun of me because I was always on the move, and when I did sit down to "read," it really meant I was taking a nap. (To this day, my family jokes about Dad going to "read" for a while.) But rest, like exercise, is a valuable wellbeing practice—we don't need to hide it, give it code names, or be ashamed of it.

Of course, rest can also be hard for people with busy lives caring for others, working, taking care of daily chores, and just getting everything done. Rest and relaxation are critical to personal and physical wellbeing; however, I urge you to prioritize them just as you would any other health practice. You can pursue relaxation without feeling guilty. Adding more quality rest into your life is a powerful behavior change to lead off your wellbeing journey.

There are several ways you can prioritize rest and sleep. First, evaluate how you spend your free time and consider how relaxing those activities truly are. For instance, scrolling through your phone to check news, memes, and social media can be detrimental to sleep, especially in the evening. Not only is the influx of competing ideas mentally stimulating, but the blue light emitted by your screen also affects your brain like sunlight: It keeps you awake just when you want to be drifting off to sleep.[2] Instead of scrolling, switch your notifications to sleep mode and choose a more intentional, calming activity. My personal favorite is reading a book in bed. I usually manage about three pages!

There are many research-supported "sleep hygiene" strategies that can help you achieve quality rest. In addition to limiting screen time before bed, you can try the following:

- Dim the lights before bedtime and use blackout shades.
- Maintain consistent sleep and wake schedules.
- Limit alcohol and caffeine intake.
- Use a sleep tracking app.
- Keep pets out of the bedroom.
- Incorporate physical activity during the day.
- Practice calming breathing techniques before bedtime.
- Put your phone on sleep mode, or consider leaving it outside your bedroom entirely.
- Keep your bedroom cool.

Try implementing one or more of these behavior changes and see how it goes; you can add more until you've built a habit of prioritizing, and achieving, good sleep.

Clinical problems affecting sleep are real. If you try some or all of the above changes to your sleep hygiene and you're still not feeling rested, it's worth seeing your doctor. A condition known as sleep apnea occurs when breathing stops and starts during rest due to various respiratory and structural issues. The resulting lack of oxygen can be quite serious, causing daytime fatigue and even leading to heart attacks, brain damage, and other issues. Signs of sleep apnea may include always feeling tired no matter how much sleep you think you're getting and/or a partner who mentions that you snore loudly or seem to stop breathing in your sleep sometimes. The good news is that sleep apnea can be diagnosed and successfully treated.[3] Asking your doctor about sleep apnea can be a wise thing to do as you look at your overall sleep situation.

CHAPTER 4

You Are How You Eat

Many books, articles, podcasts, and presentations have been created about proper nutrition. While educating people about which foods and ingredients are best certainly has its value, I believe most individuals generally know when they are eating well and when they are not. Our culture is filled with that information. There are many popular diets: Some primarily profit the diet companies, while others are regarded as reputable clinical protocols. In the older wellness paradigm, we are expected to avoid calories, carbs, and similar items. This mindset often cultivates a sense of scarcity.

However, research indicates that few people can maintain these recommendations over time. Most return to their previous eating habits eventually.[1] The "maintenance" aspect of the equation is lacking. Dieting, in general, doesn't work, at least not in the long term.

Instead, we're learning that a shift in mindset toward wellbeing—and the behavior-change principles I call awareness, skill building, and maintenance (see Chapter 31 for more details)—can go a long way toward helping us eat in a healthier, more positive way.

The wellbeing research about eating boils down to a few simple principles. First, eat modest portions, enough to feel full—but no more. Typical American portions are larger than in other countries. Our serving sizes have grown dramatically over the years, with Big Gulp sodas, jumbo popcorn, Hungry-Man frozen meals, giant plates at restaurants like The Cheesecake Factory, and more. The point is that we probably just eat more than we need in order to feel satiated.

Make a habit of listening to your body, eating more mindfully, and stopping when you're full. One of the best practical ways to start this is to take your time and pay attention to each bite while eating. This is something you probably do naturally when you treat yourself to a nice restaurant meal. Chances are that you look at your food, smell it, eat more slowly, consider the ingredients, and generally savor the experience. As you linger over the fancy meal and wait for the next course, your body and brain have a chance to synchronize. The stomach needs time to signal the brain to stop eating when it's full, so eating at a slower pace not only allows you to enjoy the meal but also can prevent overeating.

Day to day, many of us eat while watching television or scrolling through our phones; we eat quickly and barely pay attention. Instead, try taking a moment to breathe and look at your food before taking a bite. By being more present during meals, you will have fewer second helpings, feel more satisfied, and enjoy the experience more.

Another major principle of eating for wellbeing offers guidelines about what to eat. Don't obsess over nitpicky rules; strive for a primarily plant-based diet with less red meat and poultry. Prioritize colorful plates of food such as orange carrots, green peas, red tomatoes, brown rice, and pink fish. The Mediterranean diet is one example of a colorful, plant-centric way to eat, and research shows it supports positive outcomes.[2]

Again, you don't have to change everything overnight, and you're allowed to make it fun. If you're a hardcore steak lover, you could try a Meatless Mondays challenge, eating plant-based meals just one day per week, and go from there. The wellbeing approach to eating is one of an abundance mindset. Eat lots of salad and veggies, whole-grain foods, and you can even have a glass of wine occasionally. Enjoy, and think of Italy or Greece—home to the Mediterranean diet!

CHAPTER 5

Mind Your Vices: Tobacco and Alcohol

If you have a vice, it's likely either smoking, drinking, or both. Nearly 40 million adults in the United States still smoke cigarettes,[1] and almost 173 million (about 70% of the population) drink alcohol.[2] [3] The health consequences of these products have been well documented for both users and those around them.

First up, let's talk about tobacco. It's highly addictive and heavily marketed in various forms, from traditional rolled cigarettes to electronic vapes. The wellbeing benefits of quitting are immense, extending beyond the obvious boosts to health: food tastes better, it's easier to breathe, you smell better to others, you save money, and you no longer have to structure your days around an addiction.[4]

The good news is that there are highly effective tobacco cessation programs that integrate medical nicotine replacement with behavioral therapies. There's no judgment in this book, but this is a significant opportunity to make a real impact on your life.

Next, let's take a quick look at liquor. Humans have been consuming alcohol in its many forms for centuries. There are numerous studies on the pros and cons of alcohol consumption. We know there are tremendous individual differences in how people metabolize alcohol, as well as genetic predispositions to become addicted. Some studies clearly document the negative biological impact that alcohol can have on individual health, such as an increased risk of cancer.[5] However, other research reports beneficial effects of alcohol consumption, especially when done in moderation and within a cultural context.[6]

The key is understanding your personal experience and relationship with alcohol to determine what is best for you. As noted above, moderate consumption can be conducive to health and wellbeing for some people. For others, living without alcohol feels healthier and is the right choice. While tobacco is unequivocally harmful to your health and those around you, alcohol occupies a gray area that may change over your lifetime. Personally, when it comes to alcohol, I prioritize quality over quantity.

CHAPTER 6

Let's Get Physical

In the old paradigm of wellness, physical activity was all about cardiovascular workouts, pumping iron, and pushing hard because "No pain, no gain." By contrast, the wellbeing research on this topic says to "Be consistent, be social, be outside." Make a practice of walking outside every day, enjoying physical activities with friends, carrying your own groceries or gardening tools, and so forth. These simple activities can have major benefits.

Part of my personal wellbeing involves exposing myself to new experiences. As my wife says, "We can't let our worlds get smaller as we age." One way we try to keep our personal worlds from shrinking is to travel. Our travels have taken us to Sardinia, one of the five Blue Zone locations with the highest density of centenarians in the world. The Blue Zone researchers have identified key drivers of longevity, including movement, eating wisely, connecting socially, and having a wise outlook.[1]

As we traveled the countryside, I saw examples of these principles everywhere. My favorite was the day my wife and I were in the highest, most ancient part of the city of Castelsardo. It has steep stairways and streets too narrow for cars. An older woman and her husband were dropped off from a car at the gates of the city and began a trek with groceries to the inner city. As I watched the couple climb the many stairways that wind their way through Castelsardo, the husband patiently waiting for his wife at the top of each flight, I couldn't help but be impressed. I appreciated his patience and her persistence, but more than anything, I knew that this was nothing extraordinary to either of them. This is just what people do.

It reminds me that wellbeing isn't a program or a product. It's just what we do and who we are.

In my 20s, I had plenty of free time, which I spent at the beach playing volleyball, surfing, and hanging out with friends. One woman who played volleyball with us was a bit older but very fit. I asked about her routine, and she mentioned that she ran during lunch every day. At the time, that sounded really boring to me, but she explained it was her only chance each day to reconnect—with her thoughts, with nature—and to be physically active, away from all her responsibilities. That changed my perspective on running. As I've mentioned, I traveled almost every week for 20 years for my job. One of my favorite things was watching children run down the vast terminal corridors in airports around the country. Their pure joy in racing through that open space was exhilarating to observe.

The lesson here is that physical activity can be a joyful and even a shared experience, and there's no one-size-fits-all way to do it. Think about what works for you, and feel free to get creative.

A friend recently told me how much he enjoys swimming because it's noncompetitive and easy on the body, and he can wear waterproof earbuds to listen to music while he swims. Not everyone is highly athletic, but simple activities like shooting baskets in the driveway or at a park, having a baseball catch, throwing a Frisbee, playing golf, skateboarding, passing a football, and kicking a soccer ball around are all ways to bring movement into your life. And they are fun! Something as easy as taking a walk with a friend around your neighborhood is a great way to get some activity in your life, be outside, and connect with others. And dancing counts too!

In addition to caring for your body in these physical ways, taking any of these simple steps will help build greater wellbeing into your day-to-day life and environment.

CHAPTER 7

Financial Wellbeing Enriches Your Life

Financial security is directly tied to health and wellbeing. Let's face it: If you are worried about making ends meet, you are likely not thinking about drinking eight glasses of water a day or parking farther from the building to get more steps in.

Financial wellbeing can be subjective; even those who seem objectively well-off can experience poor financial wellbeing. The causes of this can stem from many things, such as a lack of discipline to spend within your means, not earning enough to cover expenses, misunderstanding financial details like car loans and credit card fees, or simply not being taught to manage their money. Many people live paycheck to paycheck, using multiple credit cards to pay bills while carrying high-interest balances and lacking more than $1,000 in emergency funds.[1]

Basic building blocks of financial wellbeing include the following:

- Track where you spend your money.
- Know how much money you have coming in after taxes.
- Determine spending priorities.
- Create a budget and stick to it.
- Expect the unexpected and build an emergency fund.
- Save early and often.
- Review your debt and pay it off as soon as possible, little by little.
- Take advantage of free money, such as employer matching in a 401(k) savings plan.

One important but often overlooked aspect of financial wellbeing is good communication about money and goals. If you are in a relationship, communicate with your partner to come to a mutual agreement on your plans. Financial concerns are a top stressor for people in relationships, so agreeing on how and where to spend is key to both financial and relationship wellbeing.

Also, consider seemingly small expenses such as subscriptions to streaming services, cable television, news apps, cell service, and gym memberships. Determine which ones you need, check for duplicates, and explore more efficient options like a group or shared plan. Use credit sparingly and contribute to your savings whenever you can.

Living within your means may not be easy, but it is wise. Our consumer society creates pressure to have nice new things, expensive cars, and jewelry. However, wellbeing and happiness are derived from things other than material goods. That's what this whole book is about!

The road to financial wellbeing is a worthwhile journey, but it can be long, complicated by systemic factors, and specific to each person or family. The chapter on behavior change can help you get on the right track, starting with clarifying your purpose. From there, you can take some initial actions to build your skills—and therefore your confidence—when it comes to money. Identify what you need to know and start learning step-by-step. There are many widely trusted books, podcasts, and programs on money management, and you can also often find free or low-cost classes and workshops through reputable local community organizations.

Keep your purpose in mind, take small steps consistently, remember your iterative mindset, and savor your successes along the way. You can get there. In time, you will figure out what works for you in terms of managing your finances and spending.

CHAPTER 8

Make New Friends, But Keep the Old

I have some friends from my childhood whom I have been meeting for 20 years in Santa Barbara, California, for a long weekend of cycling. As we gather at our traditional dive breakfast spot at the beginning of the trip, it takes maybe three minutes before we're all doubled over in tears, laughing at some silly comment. It feels so good to be together again and feel the comfort that only old friends can know: the coded language, the anecdotes we can recall with one word, and the constant heckling and roasting of each other.

There are at least two different types of social connections. With close friends and family, you have a deep connection. With work colleagues and people in your community, you have lighter ones. Both support health and wellbeing. We are all too familiar with the pain of social isolation that COVID brought to the world. We quickly discovered that we are social animals. Even my introverted friends realized that connecting with others was important to them. We even feel the absence of the lighter connections. Recognizing and acknowledging the same checker at the market or barista at the coffee shop has an impact. These small, regular connections are comforting and important, as are the deeper, lifelong ones to friends and family.

Another insight from social connection research is that the quality of friendships and social connections you have is more important than the quantity.[1] Having trusted people with whom you can share your ups and downs is critical to your health. Knowing that someone cares about you and that you care about them is foundational to your wellbeing. The message here is not to hurry up and go make friends but to nurture and appreciate those connections you do have and be open to new ones.

Strengthening your social connections is a wellbeing opportunity that complements many of the other actions you're reading about in this book. Engaging in a shared activity is a wonderful way to build relationships. If increasing connection is something you want to explore, consider linking it to another of your wellbeing goals.

Can you exercise with a group?

Go out for a vegetarian lunch with a new pal?

Take a class both to learn a hobby and to meet new people?

Practice mindfulness with your close friends?

Deepen trust in your relationship by finally having that difficult talk about money.

The opportunities here are nearly endless.

CHAPTER 9

Time Is Your Most Valuable Asset

Do you ever feel like you have enough time to get everything you need to do at work and home done? Everyone feels the time crunch, but there are ways to address it. In our culture, it's easy to get overwhelmed by the sheer number of things we must do each day, often falling into a rut where we feel like we have no time to ourselves.

Think of time as your most precious commodity. How do you want to spend it? A schedule that supports wellbeing includes boundaries and routines to get things done, and creates space for variety. You don't have to change your entire lifestyle to reap this benefit. (And, of course, there are seasons of life, such as parenting a newborn, when it's natural to focus intensively on a tough task.) The wellbeing approach is to notice if your schedule feels too squeezed and identify meaningful—even if small—changes that give you some breathing room for what really matters.

Before I continue, here's a quick note on multitasking: You can't! It might seem like you're both listening on a conference call *and* writing emails, but you didn't really hear what was being said. I have been on so many calls where people asked repetitive questions because they weren't paying attention. We can *switch* from task to task, but there are very few tasks that we can *do at the same time*. Multitasking can be very stressful and often leads to poor performance.

Finding extra bandwidth or prioritizing how to spend your time can be challenging, but it's really a chance to embody your values. Do you cherish quality time with friends and family? Do you read to relax and learn? Do you cook to enjoy and share the process? You get to choose which activities you want to add or subtract. Resting counts! So does play.

If you're struggling to find time for activities you value, consider whether you could set boundaries in your schedule that might help. The internet abounds with tips and tricks for tackling the many tasks of modern life in an efficient way. A few of my favorites include the following:

- **Complete a one-minute task.** One of the best ways to start getting things done when you're feeling overwhelmed is the one-minute rule. It comes from Gretchen Rubin, author of *Better Than Before*, a book about forming new habits.[1] This simple advice helps you decide what to tackle on a long to-do list. Just do the one-minute tasks first. Hang up a coat. Read some emails. Clear and wipe the kitchen counter. Tidy a bookshelf. Whenever you take on a one-minute task, you'll feel a sense of accomplishment and a quick boost of happiness.

- **Create a "Sunday basket."** This tip comes from Lisa Woodruff, author of *The Paper Solution*.[2] She suggests dumping your bills, receipts, and various papers into a basket. Once a week, sort your actionable papers (those that need attention) from your archive papers (those that can be filed). The Sunday basket approach is part of a larger system proposed by Woodruff that uses three-ring binders rather than a filing cabinet. (She suggests five binders for financial information, medical needs, household reference, school items, and daily operations.) A Sunday basket is probably enough for most people.

- **Buy partially prepared food.** Buying chopped-up food and meal kits costs more, but they do save time. Buying precut fruit and vegetables can be a real benefit in that you may find yourself eating more fresh foods and seeing less food go rotten. I find I consume more fresh fruit when it's just there all cut up and ready to snack on.

I am very aware of time, almost to a fault. I'm actually envious of people who get so engrossed in whatever they do that they often forget about what time it is. "Oh, sorry I'm late. I got to talking with a friend and lost track of time." I wish I could do this and be in flow more often. (You'll learn more about the flow state in Chapter 18.)

The point is, your relationship with time requires some degree of management, given that it is a limited and precious resource.

CHAPTER 10

Prioritize Healthcare

Preventive care isn't just a wellness play—it's also a critical aspect of your wellbeing. Knowing you have a doctor you can count on, an understanding of health concepts and the healthcare system, and confidence in advocating for yourself makes a huge difference in your life. The goal of this chapter is to help you better manage your health and wellbeing instead of avoiding it or being frustrated by it.

When I was in my early 50s, I started a new job that had a wellness program. As one of its benefits, we could earn cash rewards for completing certain activities. One was getting an annual physical and having blood work done. Like a lot of people, I had managed to avoid the doctor's office my entire adult life other than occasional emergency room visits for some sports injuries. At my appointment, I felt a little sheepish about visiting a doctor when I felt perfectly healthy. After all, I didn't want to waste his time (or mine).

The doctor was quick to assure me that a boring visit is the best kind. Not only was it fine to come in without a health problem, there were also real benefits to doing so. For example, my doctor explained that we now have a lot of data about my body that we can use as a baseline for future comparisons to make better decisions down the line. After I left, I had to admit that I was glad I now had "a doc" in case I ever had a problem—no more running to the ER or consulting Doctor Google.

As someone who studied the healthcare system during my academic tenure, advised corporations on healthcare benefit strategies, and built programs and services that help people navigate the system, I want to empower you to engage with it on your own terms. Consider these insider tips on managing the healthcare journey for you and the people you care about. I suggest three major steps you can take.

Step #1: Identify and visit your "doc."

Find a primary care provider (PCP) and see them regularly for checkups. (Or at least find an office that will be your home base for medical matters.) This task may be challenging, as you want to find someone you like and who accepts your insurance, but be vigilant. A great place to start is on your insurance company's website or by calling the number on your insurance card for assistance. Ask your friends if they have a doctor they like. Take the same steps to find a good dentist and vision-care doctor. Keep in mind that these specialists are a first line of defense for spotting potential health issues and illnesses. For example, semi-annual dental visits include an inspection for oral cancer, and gum inflammation can be an indication of heart disease.

Having a trusted relationship with your care providers forms a strong foundation for navigating the healthcare system and becoming your own health advocate. Always remember, if you lose faith in a particular doctor, you are free to find a new provider who is a better fit for you!

Step #2: Educate yourself about the system (insurance companies and healthcare providers) and your benefits. In other words, become "health literate."

It isn't fun for most of us to read about health insurance, but it's better to spend a few hours learning the basics when you're relaxed rather than in a crisis. Health literacy on a personal level means having the knowledge, skills, and confidence to interact effectively with healthcare systems, whether you're mostly healthy, dealing with chronic issues, or somewhere in between.[1] Start by familiarizing yourself with basic terminology—your insurance company and doctor's office will usually also have web pages, hotlines, and even real people available whose job is to answer questions and help you learn.

You'll also want to dive into the specifics of your individual health insurance plan to understand details such as deductibles, annual and lifetime maximum spending, copayments, in- and out-of-network options, drug coverage, specialty coverage, and mental health coverage. Don't be shy; contact your health insurance provider if you have questions.

Finally, identify your nearest in-network urgent care and emergency services option and have the phone number, address, and daily hours somewhere that's easy for every member of the household to find. Increasing your health literacy may feel like a challenge, but if you break it into steps and build your knowledge as you have the time, you'll gain confidence to navigate this unwieldy system.

Step #3: Develop and practice the skills to advocate for yourself.

Now it's time to become an expert on your own health—specifically, about what works for you and what doesn't in the system. Start by getting your records organized, including details such as preventive exams, immunizations, procedures, medications, and any health issues. That way, you can accurately share information with your PCP and family members as needed. Along with these medical records, you can include documents called "advanced medical directives" that explain your own wishes for medical treatment in situations where you might not be able to speak for yourself. They let your care team and loved ones know how you want to be treated should you have a life-threatening event (like my traumatic ski accident).

Speaking of your care team, don't be afraid to ask them questions. Ditto when reviewing your medical bills. While they can be complicated and even seemingly written in code, they often contain errors or items that can be challenged or negotiated with the health insurance company or healthcare provider.[2] Further, health insurance companies tend to deny coverage of procedures as a default action, something they do first without looking at the situation very closely. You can challenge that action (and your doctor may even support you in doing so).

Aside from money matters, you can also advocate for yourself regarding the information you need, the treatment you get, and so on. When you visit your doctor, come with questions, and if you need reinforcement, bring a family member or friend. It's perfectly appropriate and acceptable to request a second opinion regarding diagnosis, treatment, or procedure options. One doctor may have a bias toward surgery or medications, but another may provide alternative options that allow you to make an informed decision consistent with your lifestyle, preferences, and values. As your own advocate, you can look for doctors who suit your needs, communication style, and values. Always remember that you are in charge of your wellbeing!

When you are in the middle of an emergency, the last thing you want to do is waste time figuring out what is open and whether they accept your insurance. Friends of mine learned this the hard way when they drove around for hours from one urgent care center to another because they assumed too much and didn't find out until they got there that it wasn't an appropriate option for them. Also, going to the nearest or most reputable ER may not be the best idea if they are out-of-network. Don't assume.

The healthcare system is complicated and can be challenging, but when it comes to the actual care delivered, America's system is second to none, as I can attest from my own accident care. The key is not to let it overwhelm or discourage you from engaging. Whether for preventive health issues, chronic condition care, or acute problems like a sprained ankle, knowing how to navigate the system is beneficial for your foundational wellbeing.

HOLISTIC WELLBEING

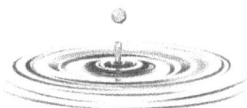

Holistic wellbeing encompasses body, mind, and spirit and involves various practices that help you live a fuller, more fulfilling life. My idea of holistic wellbeing draws from numerous expert sources that have proven goals that may seem abstract, but when implemented, can have remarkable effects on you and those around you.

CHAPTER 11

Coherence Brings It All Together

The first few chapters of the holistic section of our wellbeing buffet will consist of Gary Gunderson's five "causes of life" from his book *Deeply Woven Roots*.[1] The first is *coherence*. Sometimes, we find ourselves observing the world and trying to make sense of it all. We may come to different answers, and those answers may change with time, but they give us our sense of coherence. Coherence is an intuitive awareness that our life and world are part of a story that makes sense or has some kind of order.

In 2020—during COVID, civil unrest, political extremism, and rapid climate change—I found myself struggling to make sense of it all. This confusion took a toll on my wellbeing and that of many people around me as well.

Was that true for you? Can you think about another time when you lacked coherence?

Global political and environmental situations, along with more local or personal issues like a death in your family or community, can all contribute to a lack of coherence. How we make sense of these seemingly incoherent, unjust events is deeply connected to our wellbeing. People thrive when they experience a sense of order and understanding in the world. Questioning, exploring, and seeking a personal understanding of life's meaning are fundamental activities for developing a sense of coherence. Art, science, and religion provide ways for us to interpret a seemingly chaotic and, at times, unfair world. Having core beliefs rooted in faith or spiritual traditions, science, nature, or humanism can help ground us.

When circumstances appear disordered and chaotic, how do you cope? One approach is to talk it through with those close to you. Gain additional perspectives; learn how others make sense of situations. Also, stay grounded in your appreciation of what makes sense to you in the moment, and practice optimism that clarity will emerge in the future.

Your sense of purpose is a critical element of wellbeing and may also support your sense of coherence. Purpose is foundational to both behavior change and overall wellbeing, so I'll return to it throughout this book. There are two types of purpose to consider.

- **Life purpose:** This is the transcendental purpose that connects to something greater than yourself. It is linked to your values and beliefs about your effect on the physical and social world. While this may seem grandiose, the idea of a purpose greater than yourself leads to important questions: How can I help others? How can I improve the environment? How can I live up to my spiritual or religious beliefs? Purposeful answers to such questions are powerful motivators and core sources of wellbeing.

- **Situational and goal-oriented purpose:** For example, "I want to have healthier gums" is a situational purpose that could motivate more flossing. A situational purpose can be supercharged, however, by connecting it to a transcendental purpose. *Why* do you want healthier gums? The answer could be that this means better health and greater energy, which in turn will enable you to fulfill your purpose of helping others.

There are many ways to identify your transcendental purpose. You could start by thinking about who matters most to you. Often, people change because of others they love and care about. They want to be better parents or role models, be there for their partners, give back to their community, or live a full life with friends. It's hard to do any of that if you have low energy, jittery nerves, or a pessimistic outlook.

You can also think about what inspires you. One clue is the image you have on your phone lock screen and computer background. Are there particular quotations? Are there pictures of your kids, pets, travel, or friends? Those might say a lot about you and your purpose. Another clue is where you make charity donations or volunteer. What organizations do you resonate with most? Where and how you engage in your community can serve as a reflection of your purpose.

Dr. Victor Strecher discusses the research on purpose in his book, aptly named *Life on Purpose*.[2] This topic is personal to him, as he needed to discover his sense of purpose following his daughter's death. As a professor, researcher, and father, he explains that his purpose is to teach every student as if they were his own daughter.

Here are some more questions to ask yourself as you think about your purpose.

- Who relies on me?
- What was I passionate about as a child?
- If I didn't have a job (or other responsibilities), how would I choose to fill my hours?
- What activity makes me forget about the world around me?
- What issues do I hold close to my heart?
- What's on my bucket list?

Related to purpose are your values. Values can be loosely grouped into two categories: self-transcending and self-enriching.

- **Self-transcending values** include showing empathy, compassion, and support for the needs of others; creating and contributing to something larger than yourself; being truthful and open; committing to continuous personal growth; and maintaining mutually supportive and caring relationships.

- **Self-enriching values** include power, status, wealth, possessions, physical attractiveness, popularity, admiration, and prestige.

Self-transcending values, in particular, are associated with greater wellbeing and fulfillment.[2]

What are your self-transcending values?

Having clarity on those values that go beyond personal benefit reveals your deeper purpose and supports healthy behavior change and better social and emotional wellbeing. Please don't get discouraged if this sounds too lofty for you!

I was telling a friend about this, and she shook her head and said, "I'm not able to create world peace or solve the global climate crisis. I just care about my pets, my friends, and my garden. I guess that's not enough."

That's a common misconception. Your purpose doesn't need to be some grandiose vision of world peace. Your family, friends, and community are great places to start. And, by the way, your values and purpose may change as you grow. They might shift as you age and move through different life cycles. They're your own personal life guide, evolving with you.

Purpose is more about guiding your own behavior, while coherence is about feeling that the world around you makes sense. Still, the two are often related. For example, if you believe your purpose is to help others, but you're experiencing a lack of coherence, consider how your personal mission can give meaning and structure to seemingly chaotic events. Perhaps your own experiences of grief can deepen your compassion for others' grief, so that someday in the future, you'll be better equipped to support others going through something similar.

My recent experience with trauma has helped me relate to others in similar situations. If your personal mission is to spend your whole life learning and growing, then every experience, no matter how random, offers a chance to become a little curious and grow a bit more.

CHAPTER 12

Making New Connections

Gunderson's second cause of life is *connection*. Previously, I talked about social connection as a core aspect of foundational wellbeing, and now I want to revisit it in the context of holistic wellbeing. It's just that important! Being open to new connections and deepening established ones are profound and valuable.

I previously mentioned that I enjoyed a trip to Sardinia. What I didn't tell you was what brought me there. Spoiler alert: It wasn't Blue Zones research, at least at first. On a prior trip, this time to the Galapagos archipelago, my wife and I were on a cruise with a total of 30 people. This was our first group travel excursion, and, frankly, although we were open to the new experience, we were prepared to keep to ourselves.

To our complete surprise and delight, we found deep connections with those on the trip. The bonds were formed from a combination of the culture the captain created with his crew—which was centered on mutual respect, equitable work, and pride and purpose—and the culture we guests created by sharing meals, adventures, eye-opening education, appreciation of nature, and laughter. We hit it off with one group from the East Coast of the United States. After many shared exploits (and yes, a cocktail or two), we found ourselves making new friends! Really? At our age? We hadn't expected that. These new friends happened to be planning a trip to Sardinia. Because we'd made a great connection with them, there we were, joining them for their next adventure.

This experience provides some clues to the subtleties of human connection. At the core was the fundamental way people interacted with one another on that cruise. Both the crew and the guests practiced patience, supportiveness, inclusion, and compassion. Everyone was open to the idea of new experiences.

Connection is both a mindset and an activity. If you approach situations in your life with a "connection" attitude, the results may surprise you. You might find yourself in Sardinia, or you might find yourself joining your local historical society or starting a weekly game night with your next-door neighbors. Connections don't have to mean international travel to have positive benefits. Deepening your bonds with people close to home will keep your world from shrinking.

CHAPTER 13

You Have Agency

Agency is the third cause of life according to Gunderson. It's your ability to make choices and take actions, and your power to steer the direction of your life. Agency can be very challenging for many people because our world has so many circumstances beyond our control. Many global, local, and personal issues might seem overwhelming, unfair, or uncontrollable. So let's be clear: Having agency doesn't mean you're all-powerful! Instead, it's about having a sense of accountability, doing what you can do within your own context, and finding the insight and energy to act. When you have agency, you recognize that you can make choices. Although your options may be limited, some choice always exists. Identifying the decisions you *can make* is a powerful way to get in touch with your sense of agency.

During the fires in Pacific Palisades and other parts of Los Angeles in January 2025, my daughter, who lived in the area, was frightened and confused by this seemingly random act of nature. She felt helpless, as if she lacked agency. However, being part of the social media generation, she quickly turned to fundraising within her network to purchase emergency supplies and essentials for those displaced by the fires. She managed to regain some control over the situation, build connections, and satisfy her desire to help others. This helped her feel accountable and good about exercising some agency in an otherwise uncontrollable circumstance.

Let's look at some examples of choices you have in situations that may feel overwhelming. Suppose you feel like you lack agency when it comes to money because saving enough to buy a house seems completely out of reach. You still have the power to educate yourself about finance, set a savings goal that feels realistic, and start taking baby steps toward that goal (like establishing small automatic payments to a savings account). Exercising your power in little ways is still impactful! The sense of agency you cultivate is valuable on its own and may also grow over time.

If you're facing a situation you can't change, consider new ways to iterate and adapt to it. How can you get clever and make adjustments that improve your life overall?

For example, when I was younger, I took the bus to school. I couldn't change when the bus came, but I could control when I got up, how much time I gave myself to eat breakfast, and when I left to walk to the bus stop.

Paradoxically, choosing to accept an inevitable circumstance can also be an empowering act of agency. The famous "Serenity Prayer" asks a higher power to grant each of us "the serenity to accept the things I cannot change, the courage to change the things I can, and the wisdom to know the difference."[1] When confronted by something you can't change, can you *choose* to meet it with serenity—or another attitude that feels wise and authentic to you? If you practice being curious, flexible, and creative, you'll find that there are ways to find your agency even in the harshest or most challenging circumstances.

CHAPTER 14

From Generation to Generation

I'll introduce Gunderson's fourth cause of life with a story. As a freshman at the University of California, Santa Cruz, I lived in the redwood forest, connecting with nature and cooking for myself for the first time. Santa Cruz has a reputation as a bit of a hippie, crunchy, granola-eating place, and that was definitely true in the 1970s. Part of that culture was sharing food, especially at potluck gatherings. I was a starving student on a tight budget, buying cheap, processed food and meats.

It was about that time I came upon a book called *Diet for a Small Planet* by Frances Moore Lappé.[1] Among other things, the book explored the inefficiency with which we produce and consume food. The example that stood out for me was that it takes 20 times the amount of energy to generate protein from a cow as it does to produce the same amount of protein from plant-based products like tofu. For me, this was a profound realization: By eating animals, I was being careless with the environment. I decided then and there that I had eaten more than my fair share of meat, and it was time to preserve our resources for future generations. To this day, my vegetarianism is more about environmental impact than health. (Although later in life, I learned about the health benefits as well.)

This understanding of how our personal behavior affects future generations—and our own connection to prior generations—is known as *generativity*. It's the quality of knowing our relationship to those who have come before us and those who will come after us, and the benefits we can pass on to them. Generativity often comes with adulthood, as we begin recognizing the impact of prior generations and sense our own power to improve the future.

There are many ways to feel a sense of generativity. Environmentalism and other forms of political activism certainly accomplish this, because they're ways of speaking up for a better future. Additionally, you can do things like save and share family recipes that represent your culture and identity. Offering books and personal or community stories to younger generations is a great way to transmit your knowledge and values. Humans are storytellers, and sharing our stories with others is ingrained in us.

What do you believe would benefit the next generation—and those that follow—and how can you act on that belief? Asking these questions is how you awaken to generativity.

CHAPTER 15

Live in Hope

*H*ope is Gunderson's fifth cause of life, and it's such a common theme in wellbeing research. But what is it? At one point in my career, an organization where I worked made a concerted effort to create a positive culture. As part of that effort, they held three-day training events designed to provide personal insights. During a discussion on accountability, they introduced a tool called the "accountability ladder." This ladder indicated that blame, judgment, *and hope* were signs that a person was not taking accountability. The trainers explained that "sitting in hope" is a way of appearing to act when you are not actually doing so. To them, being hopeful meant irresponsibly wishing for a situation to improve without making any effort to help.

So even in my field, hope has many meanings, and it can be mis-understood. Let me be clear about what hope means in this book. First, hope and positivity (which you'll explore more in Chapter 29) are related concepts, yet they differ in important ways. Both can be powerful forces for optimistic thinking and resilience, yet they operate differently in terms of focus, scope, and application. Positivity is more general. It's a habit, which can be strengthened, of noticing and appreciating the good things around you, whether they're big or small. Positivity encourages us to look to the future with a generalized sense of optimism, believing that things may get better or turn out all right.

Hope, in contrast, is more specific. It's a feeling or desire for a particular outcome combined with the belief that such an outcome is possible. It often entails a sense of expectation and the motivation to work toward achieving a specific goal. Hope involves having a clearer vision for the future and believing that you can attain it, even if it requires effort and the overcoming of obstacles.[1]

Gunderson explains that hope enables us to take significant risks for a future we can visualize and believe is worth pursuing. In that sense, it is empowering, motivating us to take action.[2] Notice how this is directly opposite to hope's role in the "ladder of accountability," where it was supposedly an excuse not to act! The hope that supports wellbeing, the kind I'm discussing in this book, inspires us to act.

Research supports Gunderson's view. One study suggests that hope has two key components: agency and pathways.[3] Agency, as you learned earlier, means you have some belief in your ability to initiate and sustain actions toward a goal. Pathways, in this context, are your plans or strategies to reach that goal. Put the two together, and you have a sense of hope.

Hope might be centered around personal goals, relationships, or specific life situations. It relates to our sense of purpose and coherence, too, because hopeful goals often help us feel like we're acting on our values or giving our lives meaning. When you have hope, you're more likely to take actions toward purpose-giving, life-enriching goals.

Famous chimpanzee expert Jane Goodall offers some wonderful ways to connect with this kind of motivational inspiration in *The Book of Hope*.[4] I have wondered how a person who has devoted her life to animal protection and conservation stays hopeful in the light of seemingly intractable challenges facing the wild world. Goodall points to four things that give her hope.

- **The amazing human intellect:** Our minds can be pathways to better outcomes. Advances in technology enabled by our intellect are mind-boggling and offer the promise of unforeseen solutions to problems that seem insurmountable now.

- **The resilience of nature:** I can attest to this. I live on the California coast, and only a few years after devastating fires, we saw the forest bouncing back. Nature has a pathway to recovery if we allow it.

- **The "power of young people":** Each younger generation brings new agency, energy, and passion to the pressing issues of the day.

- **The "indomitable" human spirit:** Think about the amazing accomplishments of humankind, from landing people on the moon to running 100-mile races to providing help to those in need. We can be quite an amazing species.

What gives you hope? How do your sources of hope help you visualize goals and see pathways to achieve them?

CHAPTER 16

Cultivate Resilience

Our buffet now moves on from Gunderson's causes of life to other aspects of holistic wellbeing identified by other experts. Richard Davidson's research, as outlined in his book *The Emotional Life of Your Brain*,[1] has put a spotlight on resilience, generosity, and attention, and we'll look at those in the next few chapters.

Resilience is the ability to bounce back from challenges and setbacks. Resilience is supported by having a clear purpose (which helps you understand that what you're doing matters, even when it's hard), strong connections with other people (who can back you up and offer you care and comfort), and a hopeful outlook (which enables you to visualize a better future even when things seem challenging).[2] You can strengthen your resilience by practicing the iterative mindset covered in the behavior-change chapter, working to see failures as opportunities to iterate and figure out new plans.

One note of caution about resilience efforts: Sometimes, promoting individual resilience can avoid or miss a root cause of an issue or "blame the victim," especially in the workplace. Yes, people need to be able to do more work as organizations make changes, but let's recognize that the most resilient employee can't sustain doing the work of two or three employees due to a reduction in force, for example. As you strive to become more resilient, also notice stressors in your environment that might be a drain on your reserves.

CHAPTER 17

Generosity Keeps on Giving

Once at an informal business dinner, someone posed this question: "How do you pay it forward?" The range of answers was fascinating—and, frankly, intimidating. Some of these people were really saving the world! At least, that's how it seemed at first. Then I remembered that generosity doesn't have to be flashy to be real. Volunteering, mentoring, and improving the environment are all generous acts. So are everyday gestures of kindness, compassion, and courtesy. Ultimately, *generosity* is a way of life that includes sharing and support of others.

"But what's in it for me?" you might ask. Of course, generosity and compassion are ethically important values that we should all cherish, but why discuss helping others in a book about helping ourselves? Surprisingly, research shows that when we are compassionate and generous, it not only helps the other person—it makes us feel better, too. One study, for example, revealed that spending money on others gave the spenders a bigger happiness boost than getting something for themselves. Being generous improves our own wellbeing.[1]

There are many forms of generosity that are not about financial or physical contributions. For me, the spirit of compassion is embodied in the Hawaiian word *kokua*. For many tourists in Hawaii, the simple translation of kokua is "cooperation." However, the more nuanced meaning of the term is "to help without being asked." There is no need for reciprocation or reward; people simply value being helpful as part of their nature.

My first job after earning my doctorate was as a faculty member at a cancer research center affiliated with the University of Hawaii. My public-health work involved spending substantial time closely collaborating with members of the community. To my surprise, the most remarkable aspect of living in Hawaii wasn't the crystal-clear water, great surfing, vast sky, or diverse landscape—it was the people and the culture. The concept of kokua ensured that everyday acts of generosity were prevalent.

Think about how you are generous with your time, words, actions, and even things you treasure. Since my introduction to kokua in Hawaii, I now look for small opportunities to be helpful without being asked: I might slow down so the person in front of me has time to gather themselves at the checkout line, give a service worker a compliment (in addition to a tip), help someone with their luggage boarding a plane, pick up trash on a trail, and make the effort to be inclusive. These seem like common kindnesses and courtesies, yet they are also acts of generosity and sharing. They need no external recognition; they are part of your spirit and mindset.

CHAPTER 18

Pay Attention!

*A*ttention is rarely ever discussed in the context of wellbeing unless it is viewed as self-awareness or mindfulness. That's how researcher Richard Davidson approaches it. Focusing attention on the present moment allows us to avoid multitasking and give our brains a break from overthinking. (You'll learn more about this in the mindfulness chapter.) For now, I want to discuss two other next-level kinds of attention: paying attention to others and entering the kind of attentive state that is called "flow."

First, focusing on your attentiveness when interacting with others can significantly impact the strength and quality of your social connections. Do you notice if someone is having difficulty speaking and might need a glass of water? Or if someone requires assistance with their chair?

In particular, listening to others is a key attention behavior. How you listen is an indication of how you remain present in the moment. For example, we might not be listening well when someone is lecturing us. And how many times have you heard someone tell a story, but all you're really doing is waiting for them to finish so you can tell *your* story? My dad used to call this a "can you top this" listener. Of course, being the smart, clever, helpful people we are, we often listen with the goal of providing an answer or solution to the problem.

The truth is, though, that *simply listening* is often the most generous and rewarding thing you can do. Many times, people don't want a better story or a clever answer. They just want your attention—they want to be heard. So there's no need to give a solution—just be there and listen. That's what builds the connections that support your wellbeing.

In my opinion, the highest form of listening is listening for under-standing. When you do this, you might use phrases such as "Let me see if I understand what you are saying," "Tell me more," and "How did that make you feel?" It may very well be that we do have an answer or a good story, but by listening for understanding, we come to a deeper, more significant place in the conversation and, ultimately, in the relationship.

The second kind of attention that deserves a special shout-out here is flow, the state of being deeply focused in a natural way. I have a ski partner who, in a typical interaction, could be described as intense. Once, after a big day skiing in the mountains, I asked him if he was okay because he seemed so uncharacteristically calm and peaceful. His response was "All good, just in the zone."

The concept of the flow state—being in the zone—was popularized by Mihaly Csikszentmihalyi, a Hungarian psychologist, in his book *Flow: The Psychology of Optimal Experience.*[1] He describes flow as a mental state in which a person is fully immersed in an activity, experiencing a sense of effortless involvement and intense focus. In this state, people often lose track of time and feel a deep sense of enjoyment and fulfillment.

It's worth investigating what activities inspire you to enter flow—whether it's writing, coding, singing, or skiing—and making space for those activities in your life. Even your day job can offer flow states if it involves working without distraction on something you find fascinating and fulfilling. When you realize you've been in this state, take a moment to look back and savor it. Being in the zone, being present and mindful, is a part of holistic wellbeing.

CHAPTER 19

The Wonder of Awe

Having covered the ideas Davidson emphasizes, let's move to the next section of our holistic wellbeing buffet, where we find concepts that numerous experts promote. This may seem like a lot to add to an already robust set of concepts, but in a holistic wellbeing model, we want to stretch a little and offer many perspectives. And remember, this is a smorgasbord: Take what resonates with you, try it out, iterate, incorporate, and repeat.

Among the many things I love about children is their sense of *awe*. They exclaim "Wow!" to express their wonder and appreciation of the magnificence of things. Awe, as I define it, is a combination of profound wonder and inspired curiosity, and it's been shown to help us feel better in all kinds of ways. Awe gives us wiser perspectives and the motivation to learn and grow.

When I was in graduate school, I was fortunate to work with a highly esteemed and accomplished professor. Quite frankly, I was surprised he asked me to be his research assistant. When I asked him why he chose me, he said, "I need someone to keep me learning and in a curious place, not a knowing place." I guess I was that guy—maybe I didn't have all the "knowing" parts yet, but I was good at being awestruck!

We all need reminders to experience awe, especially as we get older. Our adult socialization tends to discourage us from letting ourselves feel or express wide-eyed wonder. We're taught to avoid sounding childlike or naïve. However, awe isn't naïve, and we don't need to leave it behind. In fact, awe can grow as we age.

My father-in-law, for example, was always in awe of people, technology, art, and science. He would be so excited to share some new piece of world music he heard that he would say, "Will you listen to this? How do they do it? Amazing!" He was always full of wonder and curiosity, attentive and hungry to learn more. And he was a very successful, creative, intelligent guy. His ability to feel awe wasn't a sign that he was out of touch. It was the opposite: a sign that he was always open-minded, learning, and growing.

Cultivating a sense of awe can profoundly enrich your life and expand your perspective. Here are some ways to nurture a mindset of wonder and appreciation.

- **Seek out new experiences.** Try new activities or visit new places. Exploring unfamiliar environments, whether it's seeking out a new hike or way home or visiting somewhere new to you, like a museum, can open your eyes to the world's beauty and complexity. Traveling, whether somewhere close by or far away, is also a great way to experience awe.

- **Practice mindfulness.** Once again, mindfulness pays off, this time in terms of awe. It helps you notice and appreciate the small details and experiences that might otherwise go unnoticed.

- **Spend time in nature.** This is one of my most beneficial practices. Nature supports wellbeing in so many ways! In this context, nature has the power to inspire awe through its scale, beauty, and complexity. Whether it's a grand vista or a tiny detail like a dew drop, nature can be a powerful source of wonder.

- **Learn continuously.** Expand your knowledge about the world, whether through reading, taking courses, or engaging in thoughtful conversations. Learning about new subjects can reveal intricate and marvelous aspects of life.

- **Reflect on the magnitude of the universe.** This sounds a bit cosmic but can be quite awe-inspiring. Contemplating the vastness of the universe, the complexity of life, or the interconnectivity of all things can evoke a deep sense of wonder. If you've never done this before and you're not sure where to start, search for "NASA images" online or, better yet, go stargazing.

- **Observe art and creativity.** There are many ways to be creative and, in turn, to feel inspired. Spend some time studying a painting or listening to a piece of music without distraction. Find a poem that speaks to you. Seek out an art installation or a public monument, and spend time taking it in. The skill, imagination, and emotion involved in these creations can inspire a profound sense of wonder.

- **Connect with others.** Sharing your experiences of awe with others can deepen your appreciation and help you see things from different perspectives. Conversations and shared moments can amplify the sense of wonder.

- **Practice humility.** Acknowledging that there is so much beyond our understanding can open us up to experiencing awe. Embrace the idea that there is always more to learn and discover.

- **Create space for reflection.** This can be challenging in a busy world, but setting aside time for quiet reflection or meditation can be an important source of awe. Allow yourself to ponder big questions or simply observe your surroundings with a sense of openness. If you attend religious services, they often provide opportunities for such reflection.

- **Document your experiences.** Keep a journal or create a visual record of moments that inspire awe. Revisiting these can help reinforce your sense of wonder and keep it alive in your daily life.

Cultivating a sense of awe is about being open to the beauty and mystery around you. It's a mindset that can be developed with practice and intention, leading to a richer and more fulfilling experience of life.

CHAPTER 20

Stay Open

Being *open-minded* to different people and ideas offers numerous benefits. In a wellbeing context, open-mindedness helps us expand our perspectives, maintain curiosity (if not awestruck!), and foster stronger connections with others. Valuing diversity and seeking ways to bridge differences are two effective ways to practice open-mindedness.

Diversity seems to be a buzzword these days; it's even politicized in some cases, for good and for ill. In public discourse, it usually connotes race, gender, age, and other important demographic differences. For our conversation about wellbeing, we can include those differences but also think about it more broadly. Diversity means that every one of us has a different point of view. That's certainly true, because we have different demographics and different backgrounds. It's also simply because we're all unique.

In the context of wellbeing, appreciating diversity means realizing that there's no one-size-fits-all recipe for wellbeing itself: What works for me might not work for you, and vice versa. That's why I keep emphasizing the importance of bringing your own goals and wisdom to bear on the advice I offer in this book.

Appreciating diversity also means valuing learning from other perspectives. As a professor of mine wisely pointed out, how brief would a conversation be if we all had the same point of view?

When I lived in Hawaii, I spent time with the indigenous community, promoting cancer screenings and preventive health. We got into many conversations about how to reach our shared goals. As we discussed how to improve the community's health, it became clear that neither I (with my public-health education) nor the Hawaiian community leaders (with their cultural expertise and local wisdom) had all the answers on our own. Instead, we found solutions through creative collaboration, building something much more than the sum of the parts.

As a simple example, I once distributed a research survey that I needed every participant to complete so I could evaluate the effectiveness of our program. However, the local leaders told me that the survey reminded people of a welfare form, so they felt uncomfortable filling it out. We collaborated with a local artist to make a different kind of form, which turned out to be quite beautiful, themed around Hawaiian values and imagery. I got better data because I respected the perspective of my partners on the project, and we all took a step closer to reaching our shared goal.

If we were all the same and had the same thoughts, styles, and preferences, then our conversations and energy would devolve. Instead, we are lucky to experience a diversity of thoughts, people, and cultures that leads to new growth and exciting results for everyone. The act of opening ourselves up to other people's differences—appreciating and learning from their perspectives and wisdom—enhances our own wellbeing in myriad ways. We don't devolve; we evolve!

Learning how to bridge differences is a key skill for being open-minded and appreciating diversity. Bridging differences is not typically part of the wellbeing conversation—and yet, how can it not be? Compromise and mutuality support our relationships, resilience, and generosity, and even link back to agency. Without the ability to connect with each other, our world would have even more unresolved conflict, which we all know is not good for our wellbeing. Bridging differences often starts with paying careful attention to what other people are saying (as you saw in the Attention chapter). It's easy to jump to conclusions, especially in situations of stress or conflict, but often, careful listening and open-minded curiosity will bring us to truths we didn't expect. Then, we can meet those truths with our generosity and compassion. (If you want to see a great example of all of this in action, check out the documentary *Will & Harper*.[1])

During the COVID epidemic, the healthcare system was under tremendous stress from unprecedented patient demand, lack of resources, staff shortages and burnout, social isolation, and general daily turmoil, as well as political and civil unrest. During that time, I had a hospital system CEO ask for advice about a problem in his organization. He explained that staff members were getting into direct confrontations and experiencing uncomfortable tension because some employees were wearing clothes with political messages or picking fights in the breakroom. Of course, these people were working double and triple shifts, many were isolating from their families, some were facing public harassment, and all of them faced the very real personal threat to their own lives and wellbeing from the virus.

In this hospital system, they had lost over 200 employees to COVID deaths. We can imagine things from their perspective. They weren't necessarily trying to politicize the hospital. They were exhausted and fearful, burdened by threatening stressors, and as a result, they were more reactive and less open-minded than they might have been in the past.

What should I have said to this CEO? In addition to urging him to enhance mental health benefits and improve access to therapy, I advised him to remind everyone of their shared personal and organizational purpose and values: to help people, to show compassion, and to value diversity. I proposed that they find ways to be compassionate toward themselves and each other regarding the stress they were all experiencing.

I am confident that some of those political opinions, right or wrong, stemmed from fear. Once we recognize that we are all afraid and struggling to bring coherence to a chaotic situation, we can start to bridge our differences. That doesn't imply we have to agree politically; instead, it suggests that we can approach one another with compassion, kindness, and a shared commitment to the goals we do embrace. Personally, I make it a point to respectfully engage with friends who hold differing viewpoints from mine to identify any commonalities we may share.

Like all the topics in this section, open-mindedness is a quality you can practice. Listen generously. If you find yourself rather insulated from diverse points of view, seek them out! Try listening to podcasts by people who are different from you. Read a novel about an unfamiliar culture. If you use social media, follow some folks with fresh perspectives or life experiences you don't know much about. One wonderful aspect of our interconnected world is that there are many chances to interact with new and different points of view.

CHAPTER 21

The Joy of Forgiveness

Once I gave a talk on wellbeing that focused on my gratitude practice (which you'll learn more about in Chapter 29). After my presentation, a gentleman approached me. He told me he practiced gratitude, but he also practiced daily *forgiveness*. I responded with awe and curiosity, and of course, I asked him to tell me more. As he explained it, it seemed to be a form of letting go. He used the example of being mad at his wife because she didn't do a certain household chore when it was her turn. He said in that situation, he had a choice: He could marinate in negative energy, or he could say, "No problem, I forgive her."

We often think of forgiveness as a moral duty, but this gentleman reminded me that it can also be an act of agency and mood-shifting. *And* it can build connections, bridge differences, and improve relationships. In other words, in a variety of ways, there are times when practicing forgiveness supports our own wellbeing.

Forgiveness is a complex and multifaceted concept that can manifest in several ways, depending on the context and the individuals involved. There are many forms of forgiveness.

- **Personal Forgiveness:** This is when you forgive someone who has wronged you. It involves using your agency to let go of feelings of resentment, anger, or hurt toward the person. It's often a process of internal healing and doesn't necessarily mean you'll inform the other person about it, forget the wrongdoing, or maintain the relationship in the same way.

- **Interpersonal Forgiveness:** This requires communication between two people. It involves acknowledging the hurt, expressing it, and then moving toward reconciliation. This form of forgiveness often requires understanding from both parties. It can lead to repairing and sometimes even strengthening the relationship.

- **Self-Forgiveness:** This involves coming to terms with your own mistakes or shortcomings. It's about releasing guilt or self-blame and allowing yourself to move on from past errors. Self-forgiveness is crucial for personal growth and emotional wellbeing.

- **Forgiveness in Relationships:** This form involves forgiving someone within the context of a close relationship, such as a friend, family member, or partner. It often requires deeper emotional processing and mutual effort to restore trust and understanding.

- **Forgiveness in the Context of Conflict:** In situations of larger-scale conflict, such as between groups or nations, forgiveness can be part of a peace-building process. It involves acknowledging past grievances, expressing remorse, and working toward reconciliation. This form of forgiveness is often complex and may require broader societal changes.

- **Conditional vs. Unconditional Forgiveness:** Conditional forgiveness is given on the condition that the offending party meets certain criteria or shows genuine remorse. Unconditional forgiveness, on the other hand, is given freely, regardless of whether the offender makes amends or changes their behavior.

- **Legal and Restorative Forgiveness:** In legal contexts, forgiveness can sometimes be part of a restorative justice process, where the focus is on repairing harm and addressing the needs of victims and offenders. This approach often involves mediated discussions and agreements about how to make amends.

- **Forgiveness as a Spiritual Practice:** Many religions and spiritual practices emphasize forgiveness as a virtue or spiritual goal. This often involves a deeper, sometimes spiritual, understanding where the focus is on transcending personal grievances for greater inner peace or spiritual growth.

Each form of forgiveness can play a role in healing and improving relationships, both with others and yourself.

Which forms of forgiveness feel most relevant to you? If there's a situation in your life where you'd like to practice forgiveness, consider whether it's something you want to let go of privately (like the gentleman I mentioned), something you need to discuss with the other person, or something that may require an external mediator to facilitate the process. Your morals and values may be your primary motivators, which is fitting, but if you seek that extra boost in wellbeing, I encourage you to view the forgiveness process as an exertion of your agency.

Are you doing this to shift your mood?

To fulfill your purpose?

To strengthen your relationships?

To bridge a difference?

Additionally, if your initial attempts don't succeed, maintain an iterative mindset. How can you adjust and try again?

The forgiveness process can vary widely based on individual circumstances and the nature of the offense, but it's almost always an opportunity to practice kindness toward others and yourself.

CHAPTER 22

Joy Is Contagious

You can't take wellbeing to the next level—to the holistic level— without *joy*.

It's tough to get motivated to be your best self without any joy in your life. Some people might even argue that joy is the *goal* of wellbeing, and they'd have a good case. But I still like thinking of joy as an option in your wellbeing buffet: something you can choose to intentionally practice and cultivate as part of your journey to a life of greater overall wellbeing.

To explore joy, you can ask yourself some questions.

What does joy feel like to me?

What things make me happy?

How can I savor the joys I've already experienced?

How can I invite more joy into my life?

The answers will be different for everyone, but if you want a place to start, you might ask what joy feels like in your body. Is it the excited butterflies you get at the top of a roller coaster? The deep relaxation that comes from snuggling up with a purring cat and a good book? Is it a simple sense of warmth when you smile at a loved one? Notice when you have that good feeling. Be mindful. Savor it. You might even say to yourself or the people with you "This is really joyful!"

There's probably more joy in our lives already than we take the time and attention to notice, so bringing it into conscious awareness is a meaningful practice. Then, as you get to know more about what brings you joy, you can use our tried-and-true behavior-change steps to make more room for joyful things.

"The Dalai Lama and Desmond Tutu spend a week on a retreat discussing joy." That sounds like the start of a joke, but it is the premise of *The Book of Joy*, which they coauthored with Douglas Abrams.[1] In the book, which I highly recommend, these two men share their insights on how we can bring more joy into our lives. Eight Pillars of Joy arise from their conversation, five of which we've already covered. Those five are…

- Perspective
- Forgiveness
- Gratitude
- Compassion
- Generosity

The three pillars I haven't addressed yet are humility, humor, and acceptance. Read on to look into these concepts.

CHAPTER 23

Embrace Humility

When I reflect on the people I respect most—whether in my personal life, work life, or the public domain—they tend to be humble, maintaining a sense of *humility* regardless of their accomplishments. The Dalai Lama and Desmond Tutu, two individuals who have impacted so many, were always known for being humble and grounded. Furthermore, in their book, they asserted that this humility fosters greater joy. The concept of humility relates to the idea of servant leadership, which prioritizes the growth, wellbeing, and empowerment of others. Believing that our role in society and the community is to support others embodies basic humility, the opposite of entitlement.

Believe it or not, many famous people get nervous when they have to speak in front of large audiences. Both of these men noted that they used to feel anxious when presenting to a group…until they changed their perspective. They shifted from feeling somehow different from the audience to simply realizing they are just another person, like those in the crowd, the same human being. This idea translates to the fact that when you meet another person, regardless of their point of view or differences, we all have the same desires to be happy and we all have the right to achieve it.

Humility reminds us that we are all the same in many ways, neither better nor worse than anyone else. This, in turn, helps us feel more connected, less isolated, and aware of what we have in common rather than our differences. We all experience ups and downs. We are all human beings striving to live our best lives with what we have.

Perhaps take a moment to reflect on times when you faced challenges in life and felt, in some way, less than others. These humbling moments can enhance your humility and compassion.

CHAPTER 24

The Funny Thing About Humor

One thing I learned while reading *The Book of Joy* is that the Dalai Lama has quite the sense of humor! It makes sense that he considers this to be an important part of joy. In my opinion, it's also a wonderful tool for wellbeing. And let's be clear: Cultivating your sense of humor doesn't mean you have to become a professional stand-up comic who can tell a perfect joke. It is more about laughing at jokes than performing them. It's about storytelling and about not taking yourself too seriously.

In fact, having a sense of humor about yourself is a great way to practice humility. Noticing when you screw up, commenting about it in a funny way, and letting yourself laugh about it puts things into perspective and shifts your mood from discouragement to amusement.

Humor also builds community. My father was born in Brooklyn, a very ethnically diverse community, and one way to break the tension between groups and within groups was with humor. To this day, in my family, we have a favorite joke that's kind of about this theme.

A new prisoner is eating his first breakfast in the jailhouse mess hall, when another prisoner stands up and yells a number. Everyone bursts out laughing. This happens twice more during the meal. Then everyone leaves for their cells. At lunchtime, the same thing happens. This time, our new guy asks the prisoner next to him why everyone is laughing. The prisoner explains that they have all been together for so long that they know all the jokes by number. They don't need to waste time telling them anymore. At dinner, the new guy decides to give it a try. He stands up and hollers, "Six!" There's a hush in the room. No one laughs. Awkwardly, the new guy sits down. Eventually, he asks the prisoner next to him what happened. That man says, "Hey, some guys just don't know how to tell a joke."

In my family, we all know so many jokes that whenever someone tries to tell one of our classics, someone else blurts out the punch line prematurely, and everyone laughs. Talk about a mood full of positivity and connection! That's just one example of how humor and laughter can boost wellbeing.

Cultivating more humor can brighten your life and help you connect with others. Here are some tips to help you bring more humor into your daily routine.

- **Expose yourself to humor.** Watch comedies, stand-up specials, and hilarious videos. Read humorous books and follow comedians or funny accounts online. The more you immerse yourself in humor, the better you'll understand different comedic styles and what makes you laugh.

- **Practice being playful.** Don't be afraid to be a little silly. Embrace playful behavior and allow yourself to be spontaneous. Humor often comes from unexpected and lighthearted moments. Kids laugh all the time; adults could take a lesson from them!

- **Learn to laugh at yourself.** Being able to laugh at your own mistakes or quirks can be a great source of humor. As a gesture of humility, it shows confidence and makes you more relatable.

- **Develop a sense of timing.** Pay attention to how comedians deliver their jokes, and try to practice good timing in your own stories or anecdotes.

- **Use humor to connect.** Share funny stories or observations with friends and family. Humor can be a great way to bond and create positive interactions.

- **Stay open-minded.** Different people find humor in different things. Be open to various types of comedy, even those that may not be your usual preference.

- **Be observant.** Sometimes, humor comes from the everyday and mundane. Keep an eye out for amusing details in your surroundings and everyday life.

- **Take risks.** Humor often involves taking risks and stepping out of your comfort zone. Don't get discouraged if a joke doesn't land; it's part of the process of finding what works for you.

- **Surround yourself with funny people.** Spend time with people who have a good sense of humor. Their attitude and jokes can inspire you and help you develop your own comedic sense; they'll also help you get into the habit of laughing more.

Be genuine and let your personality shine through your humor. But don't force it. Authenticity is often what makes comedy resonate with others. Humor is a skill that can be developed over time. Keep experimenting and enjoy the process!

CHAPTER 25

Accepting What Is

I've touched on *acceptance* a few times already. I noted that accepting a situation you can't change is, paradoxically, a kind of agency. It is also often a part of appreciating diversity, bridging differences, offering forgiveness, practicing humility, and more. It's important enough that it deserves its own place in our buffet of options as a component of wellbeing that you can practice.

Acceptance is fundamentally about understanding what you can control and what you cannot. It is the opposite of resignation. It is not a helpless state. It is a mindset that allows you to see reality and take appropriate action.

Acceptance is a worldview that recognizes our role in life's drama with humility and respect. This state of mind helps us put life into perspective, laugh at ourselves, and at some point, embrace life with all its ups and downs, pain and pleasure, chaos and beauty. Sometimes, acceptance requires forgiveness—for who you are, who others are, and the way the world is. You can think of it as an invitation to make peace with some things that you can't change.

Some of the classic stuff that's out of our control includes the future (we can never know for certain what our life is going to look like), the past (it's done and can't be changed), and most of the thoughts, feelings, and even actions of other people, especially adults. If you find yourself replaying something that happened 10 years ago, wondering "if only" this and "if only" that, consider practicing acceptance instead. It happened. It can't be changed. So how can you work with its effect on you today? How would you like to heal, change, or grow *now*?

Who knew that being an accepting person could bring joy? I haven't always been a fan of the phrase "It is what it is," but in an acceptance context, I get it. It means **I accept the way things are, and I don't necessarily have to change them. Instead, I can devote my energy to serving my purpose in other ways.**

One basic way to start a practice of acceptance is to keep a simple list of things that worry you, bother you, or pop into your head as you're trying to fall asleep. The trick is that the list doesn't have a single column; it has two. The first column is for Stuff I Can Do Something About, and the second is for Stuff I Can't Control. You can name the columns whatever you want (get creative!), but the idea is to train your brain to draw distinctions between things you can act on versus those you might need to accept, make peace with, and let go.

Here's an example of how this works: Suppose you're looking for a new job. Worries about writing your resume and preparing for your interview are concerns you can act on. You know what to do with those. By contrast, worries about whether the interviewers will like you or think you're a good fit are beyond your control. They go on the acceptance side of the list. Rather than obsess over how to manage other people's thoughts and feelings—since you can't—practice acceptance with those worries. Put them in perspective, have a laugh if you can, and give yourself permission *not* to spin your wheels attempting the impossible. What an opportunity!

That concludes our visit to the holistic wellbeing buffet. I hope you've found a few ideas that resonate, concepts you might explore further, and even behavior changes you might want to try. Remember that there's no universal road to holistic wellbeing. Everyone's journey will look different. You can always experiment, let go of what doesn't work, and adapt and iterate until you find what does.

EMOTIONAL WELLBEING

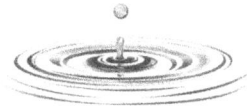

Emotional wellbeing involves understanding, managing, and expressing emotions, as well as facing life's challenges. Mental and emotional health issues are often misunderstood, so in the next chapters, you will learn strategies to improve your day-to-day experience.

Remember, you are not alone! Also, self-care is not selfish.

CHAPTER 26

Practice Mindfulness

Before we get into mindfulness, I need to address the #1 reason most people turn to ancient practices like mindfulness and meditation: stress!

Stress, in and of itself, is not a bad thing. In fact, occasional stress in manageable amounts can be helpful and productive. Researchers who study this topic refer to stressful events or situations as *stressors*. These are different for everyone. Flying in an airplane can be a stressor for one person but enjoyable for the person sitting next to them.

We react to stressors through a two-step process: appraisal and response.[1] Appraisal is the stage where we evaluate the stressor: Is it a real threat or merely something exciting or challenging? If we determine that the stressor is a threat, our bodies respond in the second stage of the process with a very real physiological reaction. It triggers adrenaline, increases our heart rate, and constrains blood flow from our extremities. This biochemical cascade is known as the fight-or-flight response. It enables us to run faster and be stronger than we normally could. That's fine in small doses (especially in a real crisis, such as fleeing a furious grizzly bear), but a chronic, ongoing stress response can lead to heart disease and other health issues.

The good news is that how you *appraise* a stressor will impact how your brain and body *respond* to it. Seeing a stressor as an opportunity or challenge instead of a threat calms the fight-or-flight response and allows us to remain in a more creative and curious mindset. Learning to shift your threat response won't happen overnight (and if you suffer from anxiety or trauma, you may want to enlist professional support), but you can always look for chances to reframe your appraisal of stressors.

For example, when the COVID lockdowns happened, many people understandably found the isolation and disruption to their schedules (not to mention the disease itself) threatening. However, the lockdowns presented an opportunity in the sense that they gave us chances to try something new, such as spending more time with family or getting creative with cooking or hobbies. People who were able to reframe working from home as a challenge or opportunity rather than a threat probably experienced lower physiological stress as a result. Basically, you can't avoid all stress—none of us can—but you can sometimes change how you respond to it, and that's a big deal.

Now that you know a bit about stress, let's talk about a powerful practice that can help you release stress and lead a calmer existence: mindfulness.

The idea of being present in the moment—being mindful—has been around for thousands of years. In the United States, the 1960s brought us the saying "Be Here Now," (coined by the spiritual teacher Ram Dass, who wrote a best-selling book by that name).[2] More recently, the concept of mindfulness has gained popularity.

When do you feel the most present in the moment, aware of your body, of your senses, of what's around you? The thing I like about mindfulness is that it's not necessarily about taking time to meditate (although that is also very beneficial). It can be as simple as taking a moment to set aside your thoughts and check in with yourself.

If you are more present and aware of all the different things you do and experience during the day, you'll be less inclined to feel trapped in a narrow rut. For example, if you wash the dishes while worrying about a conversation you had that day at work, your brain feels like you're still *at* your job, in that rut. However, if you spend even a minute or two noticing that the warm dishwater feels great on your hands, or that you're not a big fan of the smell of your soap, your brain can realize that you're *not* still at your job. There's more to life. Even if you go back to worrying about that conversation (it happens!), you've had that little break, and those little breaks add up.

As you build a habit of mindfulness, you'll train your brain to become more flexible, more open to current experiences, and less likely to be trapped in those ruts. Meditation is one of the best forms of this brain-training, but it's not the only one. Just taking that moment to be present with whatever's happening will help. Hear the sounds around you. Notice the natural environment. Really listen when another person is speaking. These are all ways to practice mindfulness.

When I was considering leaving my full-time job, I became very nostalgic. I started recalling moments in my career when I had led a great team; we all worked together and felt like we were making progress. I recalled other times in my life with friends and family that I considered great moments. And then I thought, *Wouldn't it be amazing to know the moments were great when they were happening?*

It's not that I'd been oblivious to how things were going or that I was completely unappreciative, but I couldn't help thinking how great it would have been to experience those moments more deeply at the time.

When I shared my "great moments" epiphany with a friend, he simply responded by saying, "Aren't they all great moments?" My friend's words helped me realize that *every* moment is a chance to experience life deeply, whether it's painful, neutral, or joyful. Mindfulness can apply to everything you do: eating, exercising, working, chatting, and more. Yes, you can try a formal meditation practice, but you can also set a goal of simply returning to the present moment, briefly and without judgment, throughout your day. Just take a deep breath and check in. What's happening with you right now? How does your body feel? What's your mood? What's in your heart? What's going on around you?

CHAPTER 27

Self-Care Isn't Selfish

One of the most common words in conversations about mental and emotional wellbeing is self-care. I've said this before, but it bears repeating: Self-care isn't selfish. In fact, a friend of mine, Stephanie Szostak, wrote a book called *Selfish*, which is a practical workbook to help people with their self-care.[1] One thing that stands out to me about this book is that the title is a play on the word *selfish*. I think many of us feel guilty for taking time for ourselves or believe that it is selfish to do something personal when we could be doing something for our family, coworkers, or community.

But consider this: You will be kinder and more productive, helpful, and compassionate when you are at your best—and that requires taking care of yourself. By doing so, you will better serve others and your greater purpose.

When my daughter was young, I would take early-morning runs. Both my wife and I had full-time jobs, so finding any time for myself was tricky and perhaps seemed selfish. But once I had my run, I was much better for the rest of the day at helping the family and at work.

What are some self-care behaviors you already practice? What are some areas where you'd like to feel better? Remember, while self-care can be a night out with friends or getting a massage, it's really about those activities that replenish you and make you feel good in a deep and lasting way. Self-care is very personal and may include playing or listening to music, reading or writing, spending uninterrupted time in nature, or working on a hobby. Sometimes, even cleaning the house or cooking can be forms of self-care. The key is to know what energizes and rejuvenates you, and to engage in those practices and activities that restore and maintain your wellbeing.

CHAPTER 28

Change Your Mood

As you become more aware of your moods through mindful check-ins, you may notice that they shift throughout the day. Noticing that is a great first step: It's hopeful evidence that you can often shift your mood proactively and intentionally! Recognizing your mood is powerful. Once you figure out where you are on the "mood elevator," you can share your feelings with others and begin to take steps to address them.

Mood-shifting may be as simple as noticing that you're feeling grouchy, taking a deep breath, and simply resolving to start fresh. Deep breathing regulates our mood on a physiological level, yet it's often overlooked as a key to managing stressors. Try a simple cleansing breath: Take a deep breath in, hold it for a couple of counts, and then exhale fully and slowly. Repeating that process three times can help reset your mood and awareness.

Sometimes, changing your setting can help change your mood. Move into another room or sit outside for a few minutes. One of the best things about working from home for me was my ability to spend a few minutes in my backyard between calls to reset my mood and state of mind. In fact, one study showed significant reductions in anxiety and depression when people spent greater amounts of time in nature.[1] Nature can be a bench outside in an urban setting, a walk in a park, or time in the wild. Not everyone can get to a national park whenever they want, but we can all get creative about connecting to nature or bringing it to us. For example, if you live in an urban environment, perhaps you can hang a birdfeeder on your balcony or put some plants in a windowsill.

Physical activity is also a very powerful mood adjuster. Like deep breathing, it has efficient and powerful physiological effects. You don't even have to do a full workout. If you have been sitting for a while, stand up and stretch for a minute, or go for a brief walk around your workplace. Even better, go outside and seek something natural—double up your mood-shifting power through movement *and* a change of scene. For more long-term support, regular physical activity like running, yoga, cycling, swimming, hiking, or working out at a gym all have tremendous positive impacts, not only on your physical health but also on your emotional wellbeing and, depending on the activity, even your social health. Having a regular exercise practice gives you a dependable, familiar tool to help shift your mood.

You can also do this by changing some of the stories you're telling yourself. Notice how you're narrating what's happening and see if you can find a different perspective. For example, maybe you're telling yourself a really critical and judgmental story about what's happening, like "I'm always bad at this" or "He always lets me down." What if you tried asking some open-ended "what if" curious questions instead? You might try one of these:

"What can I learn here?"

"How can I use this situation to grow?"

"What steps could I take to feel better?"

Many practices exist that are especially useful for helping us find a *calmer* mood. Deep breathing, mentioned earlier, is one. And you shouldn't overlook it because it sounds simple—it really helps. In addition to breathing, one of my favorite calming practices is called the Five-Finger Meditation.[2] You can do it anywhere—I tried it in a dentist chair, and it worked for me!

1. Start by holding your left hand out in front of you (like a STOP gesture), fingers spread.

2. Inhale as you trace up your index finger using your free hand, and exhale as you trace down it.

3. Continue finger by finger, inhaling as you go up and exhaling as you come down until you've traced your entire hand.

4. Now, reverse the process from left to right and trace from your pinkie, finger by finger, back to your thumb, making sure to inhale as you trace up and exhale as you trace down.

One of the most unusual calming tips I came across was from Cord Jefferson, the television writer who thanked his therapist on national television when he won an Emmy.[3] Mr. Jefferson said he struggled with traditional meditation, but he enjoys watching the live feed from a webcam showing the jellyfish at the Monterey Bay Aquarium.[4] Take his advice and visit the aquarium's website (see Endnotes for the link) or YouTube channel to lose yourself in the mesmerizing world of jellyfish for a brief escape during your day.

CHAPTER 29

Focus on Positivity

When my mom was 87, it was time for her to move from her home in Mexico to an assisted living facility in Nevada near my brother. She had been living on her own for several years after my father died and had built a vibrant community of friends and culture around her. She was a very independent person, and this move was a big deal. While driving her from Baja, Mexico, to Carson City—more than 500 miles in her ancient Ford Explorer—I asked her to tell me what would keep her feeling positive in her new home. She acknowledged she would miss her friends and independence but was quick to express gratitude for her new home and proximity to family.

Ultimately, she said there were two things that would keep her optimistic. The first was to learn something new every day, and the second was to remember that she would always continue to grow.

I asked my mother that question for a reason. There is very strong evidence that an optimistic outlook is highly related to wellbeing. Positivity helps to create greater resilience and promotes mental health. That said, there can be misconceptions about having a positive attitude. Positivity and optimism do not mean that you have to lie to yourself or deny that anything bad ever happens.

The fact is, as humans, we're already biased toward seeing the negative side of things. Science has shown that we're better at pessimism than we are at optimism. In other words, practicing positivity simply helps balance the scales.[1] As you learned with stressors, how you appraise your surroundings is often a choice. Do you see things positively, as an opportunity or challenge…or negatively, as a threat?

Like my mom, you can practice positivity. You can look for ways to learn something new every day, which is both fun and a reminder of the hopeful, upbeat fact that we never stop growing. Make it a point to notice small, good things during your day: Maybe another driver slowed down to let you merge, or perhaps the sunset was especially beautiful. Simply by awakening to little everyday positives that already exist, you can increase your sense of your environment as a positive place.

This ties to mindfulness and mood-shifting as well, of course. Being mindful of your focus and adjusting toward the positive helps to steer you toward an optimistic perspective. There is an old *Saturday Night Live* sketch about Debbie Downer who always gives the most negative response, no matter what people are saying.[2] We all have our Debbie Downer moments, but we can all practice seeing the positives, too.

I talked about the importance of boundaries in the context of time management in Chapter 9. Boundaries are also useful for practicing positivity. For example, our culture makes it very easy to get sucked into overconsumption of social media and an endless stream of bad news. Limiting time on social media and taking breaks from news can create more space for positivity in your life.

Finally, *gratitude* is a particular kind of positivity that has been proven to make a real difference in people's mindsets. One of my longtime friends has a great relationship with his daughter, despite them living in different towns. When I asked him about it, he told me that every day they text each other three things for which they are thankful. I loved this idea so much that I adopted it and now do the same thing with my daughter.

It's very simple; there is no narrative or judgment about the "thank-fuls," but we start most days that way. It really helps promote a positive mindset, because it motivates us to pay attention to the good things in our lives, even if they're small or silly. Plus, the practice allows me to connect with my daughter and learn about what is meaningful to her. That means that in addition to boosting positivity, I'm also enhancing our social connection! Many wellbeing practices are like that: They weave together several good things at once.

CHAPTER 30

Engage in Self-Expression

Noticing your surroundings and your mood (mindfulness) and learning to adjust your responses (mood-shifting and positivity) are powerful practices that support emotional wellbeing. Self-expression, or putting something authentic about yourself into the world, is another such practice.

A simple kind of self-expression is journaling. What you write never has to be public; it's just about putting your experiences into a more tangible form so you can more easily process them. For some, journaling involves writing about personal feelings, hopes, and desires. For others, it can be a record of the day's events or dreams. It can also be poetry, doodling, or stream-of-consciousness writing. All of these count as journaling—the goal is to make time for yourself while thinking, reflecting, and finding some peace in a busy world full of stimuli and distractions.

Talking with someone is also a vital form of self-expression. The conversation doesn't have to be about your mood or anything heavy—although sometimes that's what you need to express. Whatever the topic, a simple connection with someone else can help improve your mood and mental wellbeing. I recommend talking in person or via video chat—because being in someone's physical presence can enhance the experience—but phone calls, texts, or even old-fashioned letters are all valid ways to reach out. The goal is communication.

Be creative. Creativity is self-expression by another name. One of the most surprising things I discovered in my research was that creativity is key to human health and wellbeing. People will become depressed and unwell without the opportunity to be creative in daily life.[1] Some people have the flexibility and control in their jobs to be creative. Others are creative in home and community life.

During the COVID quarantine, I asked people what they were doing to be creative. Answers included playing music, listening to music, writing and journaling, gardening, woodworking, pottery, reading, cooking, teaching, and the list goes on.

My mom painted well into her 80s. My dad organized and listened to music. Personally, I enjoy solving problems, so collaborating with companies on how to best create and maintain a healthy culture satisfies my creative hunger.

What do you do that fuels your creativity? There are countless ways you might choose to incorporate this into your life. You could do a low-stakes craft like grabbing some markers and doodling while you're talking on the phone. Try some cool dance moves while you get dressed. Or you could find something you do already and intentionally reframe your approach to it as "creative." This is what

I did at work—recognizing and savoring the aspects of my job that fed this essential need. Participating in art, music, and hobbies can be a great way to get centered, nourish your brain, get in the "zone," and take a break from technology and daily stressors. Human beings need to be creative.

CHAPTER 31

Putting It All Together: Your New Life with a Wellbeing Mindset

I covered a lot in this book, and I hope that you are now motivated to take action with your wellbeing. My goal was not only to share some of the most meaningful elements of wellbeing but also to draw lateral connections between those elements. For example, mindfulness is valuable in its own right, but it's also connected to mood-shifting, attentiveness, and connection. Hope is related to agency, and agency matters with forgiveness. Joy connects to hobbies, humor, and awe.

You explored the significance of purpose in and of itself, and also the lateral connections it has to almost every other topic in this book—to behavior change as well as to foundational, emotional, and holistic wellbeing. There are too many more lateral connections to list: bridging differences and generosity, open-mindedness and acceptance, coherence and generativity, and more.

What new connections did you discover?

The Wellbeing Mindset

To introduce the basics of foundational wellbeing, you learned about shifting mindsets from a *wellness* to a *wellbeing* approach. Many of the core elements of foundational wellbeing connect to and support emotional and holistic wellbeing. Resting well, being physically active, and eating healthily are all connected to each other *and also* connected to other wellbeing elements such as social connection, agency, and attention. It's hard to pay attention or be physically active if you are tired. It's sometimes more enjoyable to go outside for a walk when you do it with other people. Getting in touch with nature can support you at every level of wellbeing, whether you're working on exercise, mood-shifting, or experiencing awe.

Customize your wellbeing journey. You might even want to get your doctor involved if you have medical needs—especially if you have clinical issues involving food, physical movement, sleep, or mental health. For example, if you have allergies, you may want to gain a better understanding of the gut-microbiome relationship. Due to individual differences in metabolizing foods, you might need to customize the Mediterranean diet I mentioned earlier. Avoiding or limiting gluten, dairy, and alcohol may be more or less important for you than for others. The goal of this book was to make you aware of these concepts so you could then explore them further if you want.

Think big and get creative. Going to a gym and eating kale salads are pretty healthy actions, sure—but are they the right choices for you? There are people in Sardinia walking up steep paths daily, being social, maintaining purpose, and eating well. There are people in

Laguna Beach, California, who are doing the same thing in their own way: sitting on barstools that have bicycle pedals attached so they can get some movement in while chatting and having a beer! There are people in New York City who don't give a second thought about walking many blocks to work, restaurants, or shops, and to visit friends.

Consider your lifestyle, environment, and culture. Wellbeing is personal. Everything we have covered here varies from person to person. Your mind, body, and circumstances are uniquely yours, and the wellbeing you cultivate will be uniquely yours as well: your own purpose, positivity, gratitude, and connections.

What "wellbeing" means to you can also change. Your lifestyle is a constant exercise in iterative design, throughout your life. What works for you today might need to evolve in the future. Understanding how to change your behavior by knowing why you are bothering to change (finding awareness), implementing the change in supportive ways (skill building), and having a plan to sustain that change (maintenance) are all part of the dynamic nature of wellbeing. It's not about getting started; it's about keeping going.

Collective Wellbeing

Before I wrap up, I want to say a few words about *collective wellbeing*. This book has focused on you, an individual, but we can also work together to build wellbeing for our whole communities. I have spent a career helping companies build collective wellbeing among their employees. I've seen that a culture of wellbeing supports everyone's individual journeys and makes the whole community stronger.

How can we build such a culture in our homes, communities, and workplaces?

We already have the skills we need. Our ability to connect with others socially—listening, being open-minded and compassionate, identifying shared goals and interests—is the key that unlocks collective wellbeing.

How can you practice wellbeing with others in your home and community in specific ways? Better yet, can you take the lead and make it welcoming for people to join you in some physical activity, education (related to finances or health, for example), or mindfulness practice? You can keep things simple to start; maybe you organize a family stand-up comedy night or make a pact with your coworkers to take the stairs. Perhaps you start a club or initiate an annual cycling trip with your friends.

Contributing to the greater good is also a significant way to build a wellbeing culture. Volunteering and giving back to others in any large or small way strengthens your community. There are many existing organizations that already do great wellbeing work. You can find one and support it in whatever way works for you. Some organizations focus on mental and physical health, but educational groups also offer powerful routes to greater community wellbeing.

How can you support opportunities for learning in your environment? Accessible education about money, jobs, and the healthcare system empowers everyone who participates, increasing their sense of agency and hope, as well as offering connection and support. And don't overlook ways that you might support community creativity, positivity, and awe.

For example, I get inspired by libraries. I am in awe of these institutions, large and small, that make resources and space for learning and growth part of the fabric of the community. And, for the most part, they are free and broadly accessible. What a great resource for you to use and support! I also love discovering public art: outdoor sculptures, murals, and beautiful architecture. And I find community parks to be inspiring and empowering places. The idea that we value nature and open space over commercialization is meaningful to me, so I look for ways to support local public lands.

In other words, there are many ways to get involved in your community's wellbeing. What inspires you? What inspiration do you want to bring to the people around you?

You can also contribute to collective wellbeing through your own behavior and treatment of others. In corporate settings, we often talk about the "culture" we want in the workplace and take steps to create ones that are supportive not only of physical health but also of everyone's need for clear communication, respect, and positivity. After all, even if one person is doing everything possible to address their mental and emotional wellbeing, they will still face significant challenges if the people around them are negative, unsupportive, unfair, or unkind.

Think about the "cultures" you're a part of—at home, work, or school, among your friends, or in your community. Challenge yourself to notice the unwritten protocols in your culture. Are there actions most people assume are fine—such as looking at their phones while in a conversation—that might be worth a gentle nudge to change? We all contribute to the culture around us.

Even informally, you can think about yourself as a leader and the impact you make on others daily. Think of people who create a positive culture. How do they foster it? To start, they're often great role models. So consider: Which behaviors do you want to offer to the people around you? The "shadow" you choose to cast affects the culture. Simply by modeling positivity, attention, and generosity, you can promote a connected, socially supportive environment. Further, by serving as a role model for self-care, you provide permission for others to do the same, promoting a culture where these aspects of personal growth and wellbeing are valued.

When supporting others on their wellbeing journey, try not to be critical or judgmental. Avoid the tough-love approach. Don't minimize someone's pain; avoid offering unsolicited advice or making comparisons. All people really want is for you to be there, be patient, be kind, and offer resources. You don't need to boss people around or make changes on their behalf. Instead, start by listening…then keep listening.

One final story: In the summer of 2024, my brothers and I set out for a backpacking trip on the Lake Tahoe Rim Trail. As anyone who has ever backpacked knows, being out in the wilderness for five days requires a fair amount of logistics. We are all experienced campers who know what's required—and we all have our own opinions about it, too.

Coming together with my brothers from all parts of the country, all of us in our 60s, to enjoy nature and each other's company was a wonderful experience. However, inevitably, we fell into old patterns.

We brothers form a small "culture" with its own style and expectations. One brother takes charge, offering leadership about our food, route, and logistics. Another brother optimizes, adding suggestions and modifications to our plans. Me? I tend to be a slight outlier to the group's more conventional style, but I'm also the diplomat, bridging differences and finding compromise.

As old sibling rivalries and fresh debates arose, we may have had a few spats—but our group culture was basically strong and supportive. Letting go and going with the flow became our trip mantra.

The best illustration of this dynamic happened one night around the campfire. My "leader" brother recounted a previous trip he'd taken with my "optimizer" brother. When they returned from their backpacking excursion, the leader had packed the small compact car with all their gear. When he was done, the optimizer had proceeded to unpack and reposition everything. Hearing this tale, the optimizer started laughing. The leader asked what was so funny. The optimizer replied that every night on *this* trip, he'd arranged the firewood for the campfire, and every night without fail, the leader had rearranged his sticks at the last minute. Even the leader had to laugh as the optimizer burst out, "Stop moving my sticks!"

I love this incident for many reasons, but especially because it shows how we can often have the best intentions but still end up trying to control other people instead of listening to them and supporting them. I thought, *Pretty cool.* Now, when I'm working on my own relationships or striving to improve my community's wellbeing, I ask myself these questions:

Whose sticks am I moving?

Who am I not letting have a chance to be right, to be creative, or to contribute?

How can I allow us to do this together instead of making it all about me?

Collective wellbeing is for everybody, and we can craft our cultures to support that.

And that's that! My intention with this book is to help you have a better understanding of why you should pay close attention to your wellbeing and remove the pressure from your feeling as if you have to make some momentous lifestyle change to improve it. I hope you feel inspired to embark on a journey toward greater wellbeing.

Of all the things that you read in this book, what stuck out for you? Pick an easy first step and give it a try. Figure out how to make it doable and fun. Grow and connect with others.

Serve your purpose by being well.

About the Author

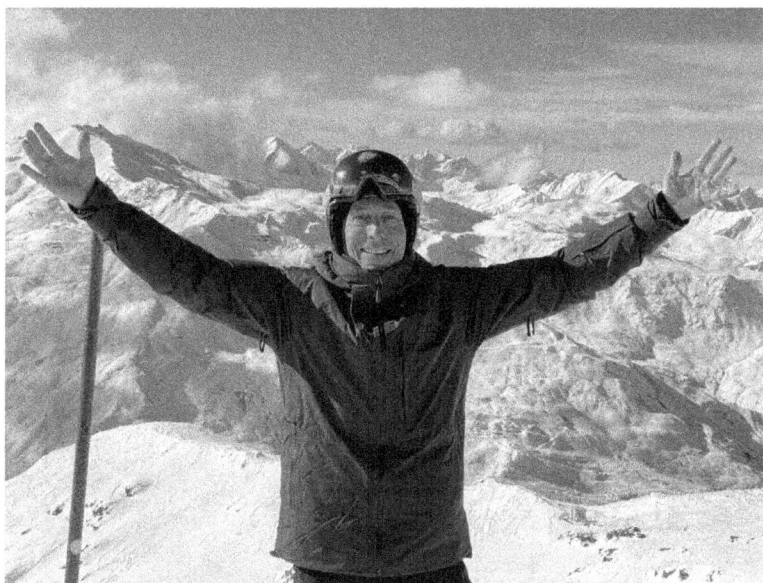

Dr. Seth Serxner brings 30 years of experience in academia, industry, and consulting to his understanding of health and wellbeing. Through his ability to translate the science of wellbeing into an easy-to-understand language and practices, he has published over 50 articles and has helped hundreds of companies and their employees live happier, healthier lives.

He spent a decade each in academia and private industry before becoming a consultant. He was vice president of research at StayWell, where he established the industry-leading market research program for developing and marketing consumer health materials and programs. He has held academic positions with the University of Hawaii Medical School, the Cancer Research Center of Hawaii, and the University of California, Irvine. More recently, he was the Chief Health Officer at an industry-leading health services company.

Seth earned his undergraduate degree in psychology at the University of California, Santa Cruz; a Master of Public Health from the University of California, Los Angeles; and a doctorate from the University of California, Irvine, where he currently studies health promotion and disease prevention.

He serves on two industry boards of directors as well as on the UnitedHealthcare Children's Foundation, which provides medical grants for families in need.

Seth lives with his wife in Half Moon Bay, California, and they have one daughter. It is no surprise that he is a runner, skier, hiker, and cyclist and will play any sport that has a ball and a net.

Acknowledgments

There is a long list of people who have helped me in my education and career without whom this book would not have been possible. Going way back, I want to thank Dr. Ralph Catalano for taking me on as his doctoral student and Peter Bergen, who took a chance on me at my first private-sector job transitioning from academia. I am thankful for the opportunity to work with leaders at T-Mobile, Lumen, Lowe's home improvement, PepsiCo, as well as many others who gave me diverse experiences and insights regarding the practice of wellbeing at scale.

Regarding this book, I owe thanks to Catherine Gregory and Nathan Joblin from Modern Wisdom Press, who guided me through the entire process and helped me develop my manuscript to launch an actual book; and thank you to Holly Moyer and Trudi Roth for being amazing editing partners.

I want to recognize my friend Alex Siskin, who gave me the notion to write a book while we were taking a long walk on the beach and then helped guide me in the initial process.

I also want to thank Jessica Grossmeier for her generous support in the book-writing process including sharing her personal experience working with Modern Wisdom Press to write and publish her book.

Last but not least, I want to thank my wife and daughter, as well as my two brothers, for their love and support for my wellbeing and my ability to complete this book.

As I mentioned in the introduction, our lives are connected to so many people in ways that we would not have necessarily planned or predicted. I feel compelled to list some of the people who have had an influence on my career and thinking. David Anderson, Paul Terry, Kenneth Pelletier, Daniel Gold, Ron Goetzel, Stephen Noeldner, John Tarbuck, Kristin Baker, Sue Willette, Howard Kraft, Thomas Murray, Chris Ciatto, Marie Schmitt, Shelly Wolf, Stephanie Szostak, Tom Chamberlain, Sushant Gupta, David Hoke, Victor Strecher, Eric Zimmerman, Cyrus Batheja, Steve Olin, Pamela Rich, and Mindy Fox.

And to my friends who put up with countless hours of me droning on during long bike rides, hikes, chairlift rides, travels, and any other chance I had about purpose, hope, gratitude, and all the wellbeing principles—thank you. You know who you are, and I appreciate you!

Endnotes

Chapter 2

1. Centers for Disease Control and Prevention. 2022. "Current Cigarette Smoking Among Adults in the United States." https://www.cdc.gov/tobacco/php/data-statistics/adult-data-cigarettes/?CDC_AAref_Val=https://www.cdc.gov/tobacco/data_statistics/fact_sheets/adult_data/cig_smoking/index.html.

2. Keep America Beautiful. 2021. "2020 National Litter Study." https://kab.org/wp-content/uploads/2021/05/Litter-Study-Summary-Report-May-2021_final_05172021.pdf.

3. Brenan, Megan. 2021. "Smoking and Vaping Remain Steady and Low in U.S." *Gallup*, August 12, 2021. https://news.gallup.com/poll/353225/smoking-vaping-remain-steady-low.aspx.

4. National Highway Traffic Safety Administration. 2021. "Seat Belt Use in 2021 – Overall Results." https://www.nhtsa.gov/risky-driving/seat-belts.

5. Levy, David T., An-Tsun Huang, Joshua S. Havumaki, and Rafael Meza. 2016. "The Role of Public Policies in Reducing Smoking Prevalence: Results from the Michigan SimSmoke Tobacco Policy Simulation Model." *Cancer Causes & Control* 27: 615–625.

6. Nichols, James L., A. Scott Tippetts, James C. Fell, Angela H. Eichelberger, and Philip W. Haseltine. 2014. "The Effects of Primary Enforcement Laws and Fine Levels on Seat Belt Usage in the United States." *Traffic Injury Prevention* 15(6): 640–644.

7. Leeabai, Nattapon, Chinnathan Areeprasert, Chanoknunt Khaobang, et al. 2021. "The Effects of Color Preference and Noticeability of Trash Bins on Waste Collection Performance and Waste-Sorting Behaviors." *Waste Management* 121: 153–163.

8. Bobinet, Kyra. 2015. *Well Designed Life: 10 Lessons in Brain Science & Design Thinking for a Mindful, Healthy, & Purposeful Life*. Idea Press Publishing.

9. Knowles, Malcolm S. 1984. *The Adult Learner: A Neglected Species*. Gulf Publishing.

Chapter 3

1. Baron, Kelly Glazer, and Elizabeth Culnan. 2019. "Sleep and Healthy Decision Making." In *Sleep and Health*, edited by Michael A. Grandner. Academic Press.

2. Haghani, Masoud, Samaneh Abbasi, Leila Abdoli, et al. 2024. "Blue Light and Digital Screens Revisited: A New Look at Blue Light from the Vision Quality, Circadian Rhythm and Cognitive Functions Perspective." *Journal of Biomedical Physics & Engineering* 14(3): 213.

3. Slowik, Jennifer M., Abdulghani Sankari, and Jacob F. Collen. 2024. "Obstructive Sleep Apnea." In *StatPearls [Internet]*. StatPearls Publishing.

Chapter 4

1. van't Riet, Jonathan, Siet J. Sijtsema, Hans Dagevos, and Gert-Jan De Bruijn. 2011. "The Importance of Habits in Eating Behaviour. An Overview and Recommendations for Future Research." *Appetite* 57(3): 585–596. https://pubmed.ncbi.nlm.nih.gov/21816186/.

2. Crous-Bou, Marta, José-Luis Molinuevo, and Aleix Sala-Vila. 2019. "Plant-Rich Dietary Patterns, Plant Foods and Nutrients, and Telomere Length." *Advances in Nutrition* 10: S296–S303.

Chapter 5

1. Center for Disease Control. 2016. *Tobacco Use Extinguishing the Epidemic.* https://stacks.cdc.gov/view/cdc/51999/cdc_51999_DS1.pdf.

2. National Institute on Alcohol Abuse and Alcoholism. 2023. "Alcohol's Effects on Health. Research-Based Information on Drinking and Its Impact."

3. Substance Abuse and Mental Health Services Administration. "2018 National Survey on Drug Use and Health." https://www.samhsa.gov/data/data-we-collect/nsduh-national-survey-drug-use-and-health/national-releases/2018.

4. Patil, Abhinandan, and Neha Singh. 2023. "Tobacco's Toll: Looking at the Long-Term Systemic Effects." https://www.preprints.org/manuscript/202307.0950/download/final_file.

5. Yoo, Jung Eun, Kyungdo Han, Dong Wook Shin, et al. 2022. "Association Between Changes in Alcohol Consumption and Cancer Risk." *JAMA Network Open* 5(8): e2228544–e2228544.

6. Poli, Andrea. 2022. "Is Drinking Wine in Moderation Good for Health or Not?" *European Heart Journal Supplements* 24(I): I119–I122.

Chapter 6

1. Buettner, Dan. 2010. *The Blue Zones: Lessons for Living Longer from the People Who've Lived the Longest.* National Geographic Books.

Chapter 7

1. Bankrate. 2022. "More Than Half of Americans Can't Afford a $1,000 Emergency Expense." https://www.bankrate.com/banking/savings/financial-security-0118/.

Chapter 8

1. Holt-Lunstad, Julianne. 2024. "Social Connection as a Critical Factor for Mental and Physical Health: Evidence, Trends, Challenges, and Future Implications." *World Psychiatry* 23(3): 312–332.

Chapter 9

1. Rubin, Gretchen. 2015. *Better Than Before: Mastering the Habits of Our Everyday Lives.* Crown.

2. Woodruff, Lisa. 2020. *The Paper Solution: What to Shred, What to Save, and How to Stop It from Taking Over Your Life.* Putnam Publishing Group.

Chapter 10

1. Office of Disease Prevention and Health Promotion. 2021. *Health Literacy in Healthy People 2030.* https://odphp.health.gov/healthypeople/priority-areas/health-literacy-healthy-people-2030.

2. Newman, Saul Justin. 2019. "Supercentenarian and Remarkable Age Records Exhibit Patterns Indicative of Clerical Errors and Pension Fraud." *bioRxiv.* doi: https://doi.org/10.1101/704080.

Chapter 11

1. Gunderson, Gary R. 2007. *Deeply Woven Roots: Improving the Quality of Life in Your Community.* Fortress Press.

2. Strecher, Victor. 2016. *Life on Purpose: How Living for What Matters Most Changes Everything.* HarperOne.

Chapter 13

1. Niebuhr, Reinhold. 1951. *The Serenity Prayer*. Oxford University Press.

Chapter 14

1. Lappé, Frances Moore. 1991. *Diet for a Small Planet*. Ballantine Books.

Chapter 15

1. Snyder, Charles R. 1994. *The Psychology of Hope: You Can Get There from Here*. Free Press.

2. Gunderson, Gary R. 2007. *Deeply Woven Roots: Improving the Quality of Life in Your Community*. Fortress Press.

3. Snyder, Charles R., and Shane J. Lopez, eds. 2000. *Handbook of Positive Psychology*. Oxford University Press.

4. Goodall, Jane, Douglas Abrams, and Gail Hudson. 2021. *The Book of Hope: A Survival Guide for Trying Times*. Celadon Books.

Chapter 16

1. Davidson, Richard J., and Sharon Begley. 2012. *The Emotional Life of Your Brain: How Its Unique Patterns Affect the Way You Think, Feel, and Live—and How You Can Change Them*. Penguin Books.

2. MacLeod, Stephanie, Sandra Kraemer, Annette Fellows, et al. 2021. "Defining the Personal Determinants of Health for Older Adults." *Journal of Behavioral Health* 10: 1–6.

Chapter 17

1. Dunn, Elizabeth W., Lara B. Aknin, and Michael I. Norton. 2008. "Spending Money on Others Promotes Happiness." *Science* 319(5870): 1687–1688.

Chapter 18

1. Csikszentmihalyi, Mihaly. 1990. *Flow: The Psychology of Optimal Experience*. Harper & Row.

Chapter 20

1. Ferrell, Will, and Harper Steele. *Will & Harper*. Directed by Josh Greenbaum. Netflix, 2024.

Chapter 22

1. Dalai Lama, Desmond Tutu, and Douglas Abrams. 2016. *The Book of Joy: Lasting Happiness in a Changing World*. Avery.

Chapter 26

1. Lazarus, Richard S., and Susan Folkman. 1987. "Transactional Theory and Research on Emotions and Coping." *European Journal of Personality* 1(3): 141–169.

2. Dass, Ram. 1971. *Be Here Now*. Lama Foundation.

Chapter 27

1. Szostak, Stephanie. 2021. *SELF!SH: Step into a Journey of Self-Discovery to Revive Confidence, Joy, and Meaning*. Post Hill Press.

Chapter 28

1. White, Mathew P., Ian Alcock, James Grellier, et al. 2019. "Spending at Least 120 Minutes a Week in Nature Is Associated with Good Health and Wellbeing." *Scientific Reports* 9(1): 7730.

2. Bell, Mike. 2010. "The Wisdom of Ordinary Children." Parallax, June 2010. https://www.parallax.org/mindfulnessbell/article/the-wisdom-of-ordinary-children/.

3. Parker-Pope, Tara. 2020. "And the Emmy Goes to … My Therapist." *New York Times*, September 24, 2020. https://www.nytimes.com/2020/09/24/well/mind/cord-jefferson-emmy-black-mental-health.html.

4. Monterey Bay Aquarium. Jelly Cam. https://www.montereybay-aquarium.org/animals/live-cams/jelly-cam.

Chapter 29

1. Steinhilber, Brianna. "How to Train Your Brain to Be More Optimistic." NBCNews.com. August 24, 2017. https://www.nbcnews.com/better/health/how-train-your-brain-be-more-optimistic-ncna795231.

2. Dratch, Rachel. 2004. *Saturday Night Live.* Season 29, episode 18. "Debbie Downer: Disneyland." Aired May 1, 2024, on NBC.

Chapter 30

1. Cropley, Arthur J. "Creativity and Mental Health in Everyday Life." *Creativity Research Journal* 3(3): 167–178.

Thank You

Dear Reader,

Thank you for taking time out of your busy life to read this book. My wish is that you now have a new approach to your health and wellbeing. I hope this book has inspired you, motivated you, and lifted the pressure off being well to embracing your wellbeing.

If you know someone who could benefit from the ideas in this book, thank you for spreading the word! Share a copy with colleagues, friends, and family. Consider writing a book review on Amazon, which will help other readers find it.

Please visit my website (SethSerxner.com) to learn more about my podcasts, my keynote talks, and other wellbeing offerings. Reach out there to let me know your thoughts about the book and how your wellbeing journey is going. I would love to hear from you!

About
Modern Wisdom Press

Founded by Catherine Gregory and Nathan Joblin in 2019, Modern Wisdom Press is dedicated to elevating conscious voices by empowering visionary leaders and subject-matter experts to find clarity, ease, and joy in writing and publishing their transformational nonfiction books.

Our values and core principles are rooted in conscious leadership, which begins with self-awareness and intentionality, awakening more fulfillment and purpose in your life and those you lead. We support aspiring authors who are here to make a positive impact, with the ripple effect benefiting not only their readers, but also their families, communities, and beyond.

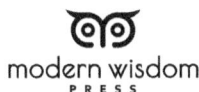

modern wisdom
PRESS

www.ingramcontent.com/pod-product-compliance
Lightning Source LLC
Chambersburg PA
CBHW032054040426
42335CB00037B/716